Neuroplasticity Explained

Alex Rossi

Copyright © 2024 Alex Rossi

All rights reserved.

ISBN: 9798337635057

CONTENTS

1 The Basics of Neuroplasticity .... Pg 7

2 Historical Perspectives .... Pg 27

3 Mechanisms of Plasticity .... Pg 41

4 Plasticity in Learning and Memory .... Pg 59

5 Neuroplasticity in Disease and Recovery .... Pg 81

6 Age and Neuroplasticity .... Pg 96

7 Technological and Therapeutic Advances .... Pg 114

8 Future Directions in Neuroplasticity Research. Pg 130

INTRODUCTION

Welcome to "Neuroplasticity Explained," your comprehensive guide to one of neuroscience's most fascinating fields. Neuroplasticity, the brain's remarkable ability to reorganize itself in response to learning, injury, and experience, challenges many of our traditional ideas about the brain. This book aims to demystify the complex concepts and intricate mechanisms that govern this dynamic process, making the science accessible and engaging to everyone, from curious novices to seasoned enthusiasts.

I want to apologize that there are no illustrations in this book, so it may be handy to have a laptop or a tablet open to view certain parts of the brain that we discuss for a better illustration.

In this exploration, we dive into the A-Z of neuroplasticity, starting with its foundational theories and moving through to the latest advancements in the field. Each chapter is crafted with simplicity and clarity, using layman's terms to navigate the depths of high-level scientific discussions. To illuminate these concepts, the book employs vivid, real-world examples and relatable analogies that connect neuroscientific phenomena with everyday experiences.

Readers can look forward to uncovering how neuroplasticity impacts learning new skills, recovering from brain injuries, and adapting to life's myriad challenges. We will explore how this incredible flexibility of the brain contributes not only to our survival but also to our capacity to develop, innovate, and transcend our limitations.

Moreover, "Neuroplasticity Explained" does not shy away from the frontiers of current research and the pressing questions that drive today's neuroscientific inquiry. What are the limits of neuroplasticity? How can emerging technologies harness this brain power to treat neurological disorders? What does the future hold for brain enhancement?

Through engaging narrative and expert insights, this book will not just educate—but also inspire readers to appreciate the untapped potential of their own brains. Whether you're a student aiming to grasp your coursework, a professional in psychology or healthcare, or simply someone eager to enhance your cognitive capabilities, this book promises to enhance your understanding and spark your fascination with the ever-evolving world of neuroplasticity. Join us on this enlightening journey to understand the malleable nature of the human brain and its implications for future innovations in science and medicine.

THE BASICS OF NEUROPLASTICITY

Neuroplasticity is not just a scientific term; it's a reflection of the brain's remarkable ability to adapt and evolve throughout an individual's life. This concept, once believed impossible by neuroscientists, underlies everything from learning new skills to recovering from traumatic brain injuries. The basis of neuroplasticity lies in the brain's dynamic potential to rewire itself—forming new connections and pathways in response to every experience, thought, and emotion. By understanding neuroplasticity, we unlock a deeper awareness of how habits form, how rehabilitation can reshape lives, and how continual learning impacts our cognitive resilience. This chapter thoroughly unpacks the mechanisms of neuroplasticity, emphasizing not just how this ability functions, but why it's essential for our interaction with the world and our personal development. As you venture through these explanations, anticipate a clear, concise exposition of how your brain is sculpted by your environment and experiences, illustrating the profound impact of our everyday actions on our brain's structure and capabilities.

Neuroplasticity rests on the principle that the brain is not fixed but is constantly being reshaped by its experiences. At the heart of this concept is the brain's ability to alter its structure and function in response to various stimuli, a capability that is paramount during learning or the recovery from a brain injury. To break it down: when we learn something new, certain pathways in our brain become active.

With repeated use, these pathways strengthen, a process known as synaptic strengthening. Meanwhile, those that are seldom used tend to weaken and diminish over time, referred to as synaptic pruning. This ability to strengthen or prune connections based on activity is what allows for the flexibility and adaptability of our cognitive functions.

During the recovery from a brain injury, neuroplasticity plays a crucial role. If a particular area of the brain is damaged, the tasks it performed may seem lost. However, other parts of the brain can sometimes take over these functions via a process called neural reassignment or compensatory masquerade, where different neural circuits rewire themselves to perform necessary tasks previously handled by the damaged area.

The scientific mechanism behind this involves several stages of neural changes. Initially, there's a rapid, yet temporary increase in the brain's plasticity, allowing neurons to form new connections quickly. Over time, as recovery progresses, the brain gradually stabilizes these connections, integrating them into regular function. This dynamic illustrates the brain's remarkable resilience and highlights the critical window immediately following an injury where therapeutic interventions can be most beneficial.

Visualizing this process can be likened to rerouting traffic in a bustling city—when the main route is blocked due to construction (the injury), detours (alternative neural pathways) are set up. Over time, these detours can become permanent paths if the primary route remains inaccessible, showcasing the brain's adaptability similar to a city's traffic system.

Understanding neuroplasticity not only shines a light on how we learn and recover but also underscores the potential for re-engineering our cognitive landscape at any age, offering hope for rehabilitation and personal development. This dynamic, continuously evolving field encourages a proactive approach to mental health and cognitive activities, with the brain's adaptability at its core, emphasizing that each interaction we have with our world is indeed shaping our brain's architecture.

Let's take a deeper look at the intricate biochemical pathways and cellular mechanisms that underpin synaptic strengthening and pruning during neuroplasticity. These processes are fundamental to how our brains adapt to new experiences and recover from injuries.

Starting with synaptic strengthening, this occurs when neurotransmitters like glutamate and dopamine play pivotal roles. These chemical messengers bind to specific receptors on post-synaptic neurons, such as NMDA receptors for glutamate, initiating a cascade of intracellular signals. One crucial pathway involves the influx of calcium ions, which activate a series of enzymes. These enzymes lead to the activation of gene transcription factors that ultimately enhance the production of proteins crucial for strengthening the synapse. This process not only solidifies new learning but also enhances the connections between neurons, making future transmission across this pathway more efficient.

On the flip side, synaptic pruning involves the removal of less active or unnecessary synapses. This is equally important as it enhances neural efficiency by eliminating weaker synaptic connections. Key players in this process include signaling proteins like the complement system, which tags inactive synapses for removal. Microglia, the brain's immune cells, recognize these tags and engulf the designated synapses, effectively pruning them away. This process is not just a cleanup operation; it's a fine-tuning of neural circuits that ensures our brains are not overloaded with superfluous connections, which can happen after brain injuries or due to neurodegenerative diseases.

The fascinating aspect is how these processes can vary between different types of neurons and brain regions. For example, in the hippocampus, a brain area vital for forming memories, synaptic strengthening is highly active, continuously adjusting the connections to store new memories efficiently. Contrastingly, in the adult cortex, synaptic pruning might be more prevalent, reflecting the need to maintain efficiency in well-established cognitive functions.

These microscopic events are crucial for the brain's adaptability and directly influence behavior. Enhanced synaptic connections can lead to improved memory and learning capabilities, often observed after consistent training or learning activities. Similarly, effective synaptic pruning can help in quicker recovery from neural injuries by reallocating neural resources to more essential or frequently used pathways.

Understanding these processes in simple terms helps us appreciate the dynamic and highly adaptive nature of our brains. It reveals the unseen world of neural interactions that shape our everyday behaviors and cognitive functions. This deep dive into the cellular level of neuroplasticity not only enriches our understanding but also highlights the vast potential of our brains to adapt, learn, and recover throughout our lives.

Understanding synaptic strengthening, synaptogenesis, and synaptic pruning is essential for grasping how our brains adapt and change in response to experiences. Let's break down these complex processes into fundamental components, making them accessible and insightful.

Starting with synaptic strengthening, this process involves the strengthening of existing connections between neurons. Think of it like a pathway in a forest that becomes clearer and more defined the more it's traveled. In neurological terms, when a signal frequently activates a particular synapse, it enhances the effectiveness of this synaptic connection. This is achieved through the increased release of neurotransmitters and the growth of receptor sites on the receiving neuron, making future transmissions across this pathway faster and more efficient.

Synaptogenesis refers to the creation of new synapses. This occurs when new experiences or learning provoke the brain to form additional synaptic connections, essentially constructing new pathways. This can be likened to forging a new trail in our hypothetical forest. Neurons sprout new branches (dendrites and axons), which reach out to other neurons, forming new synaptic contacts. This process is fundamental during early development and plays a crucial role in learning and memory throughout our lives.

On the other hand, synaptic pruning is the process of selectively eliminating less-used synapses. This mechanism is similar to pruning a bush; it helps enhance the health and efficiency of a plant, or in this case, the neural network. Pruning helps to refine neural circuits based on experience - connections that are seldom used get cut, making the overall network more efficient. This process peaks during early childhood but continues into adulthood, playing a critical role in learning and memory by removing redundant connections to streamline neural processing.

Each of these mechanisms shows the brain's dynamic ability to adapt based on interactions with the environment, ensuring cognitive efficiency and flexibility. By understanding these processes, we gain insights into the practical aspects of how learning occurs and how recovery from neural injuries can be facilitated. This knowledge not only enriches our understanding of brain functionality but also underscores the significance of engaging with varied and meaningful experiences to foster an optimally functioning brain.

Understanding the molecular and biochemical components of synaptic strengthening, synaptogenesis, and synaptic pruning is crucial for grasping how our brains adapt and change. This guide will detail each of these processes step by step, starting with the neurotransmitters involved in synaptic strengthening.

1. **Synaptic Strengthening:**
   - **Neurotransmitters such as Glutamate and GABA:** These neurotransmitters are critical in synaptic strengthening. Glutamate, for instance, binds to NMDA and AMPA receptors on the post-synaptic neuron. This interaction prompts the opening of ion channels, leading to an influx of calcium ions.
   - **Role of Calcium Ions:** The influx of calcium ions is a pivotal moment in synaptic strengthening. These ions activate a cascade of signaling pathways inside the neuron, including the activation of protein kinases that modify synaptic proteins and increase synaptic efficacy.

2. **Synaptogenesis:**
   - **Role of Neural Growth Factors:** Brain-Derived Neurotrophic Factor (BDNF) is a key player in synaptogenesis. BDNF interacts with TrkB receptors on neurons, initiating signaling pathways that promote the growth of dendrites and axons—effectively fostering the formation of new synapses.
   - **Neuron Branching and Synapse Formation:** As neurons extend their dendrites and axons, they form new synaptic connections with other neurons. This physical connection involves the assembly of synaptic structures and the recruitment of synaptic vesicles and receptors.

3. **Synaptic Pruning:**
   - **Cellular Cleanup:** Synaptic pruning is similar to pruning unnecessary branches off a tree to enhance its health

and shape. In the brain, microglia play a significant role in this cleanup process. They engulf and digest synaptic elements that are weak or unnecessary.

   - **Role of Complement Proteins:** Complement proteins label weak synapses for removal. Microglia identify these labels and subsequently remove the tagged synapses, streamlining neural communication pathways.

4. **Linking Molecular Processes to Cognitive Effects:**
   - Each of these molecular processes—synaptic strengthening, synaptogenesis, and synaptic pruning—plays an important role in brain function. Synaptic strengthening and synaptogenesis enhance the brain's ability to learn and store new information, making our memory sharper and our learning process more efficient. Conversely, synaptic pruning removes unnecessary neural connections, making the overall neural network more efficient. Collectively, these processes contribute to our brain's adaptability, function, and ultimately, our cognitive health.

This guide explicates how intricate biochemical and molecular events in the brain underpin significant cognitive functions. Understanding these connections not only enriches our knowledge of brain functionality but also emphasizes the profound impact of our daily activities and health on our overall cognitive abilities.

Age, exercise, and cognitive challenges significantly influence the neuroplastic capabilities of the brain, each affecting how the brain adapts and changes in response to experiences.

Starting with age, it is often observed that young brains exhibit higher plasticity, making them more adaptable in learning new skills and languages. As the brain ages, its neuroplasticity tends to decline, which can slow learning processes and make recovery from neural injuries more challenging. However, consistent mental stimulation and learning can help maintain and even improve neuroplasticity in older adults.

Exercise is another powerful influencer of neuroplasticity. Regular physical activity increases the production of neurotrophic factors, such as Brain-Derived Neurotrophic Factor (BDNF), which supports the formation of new neural connections and the survival of existing ones. For example, aerobic exercises like swimming or jogging not only enhance blood flow to the brain but also boost neuron health, thereby facilitating better memory and cognitive function.

Cognitive challenges play a crucial role as well. Engaging in complex problem-solving tasks or learning new skills stimulates the brain and encourages the formation of new neural pathways. This is similar to forging a new trail in the woods—the more frequently the pathway is used, the more defined and accessible it becomes. For instance, learning to play a musical instrument or solving puzzles like crosswords can significantly enhance brain plasticity, enabling the brain to remain active and agile despite aging.

Understanding how these factors interact provides insight

into the dynamic nature of neuroplasticity and emphasizes the importance of a lifestyle that incorporates regular physical and mental exercise to support cognitive health and flexibility. This outline details how everyday actions and choices impact the intricate mechanisms within the brain, promoting a lifestyle conducive to maintaining an adaptable and sharp mind.

Here is the detailed breakdown of the molecular and cellular mechanisms affected by exercise in promoting neuroplasticity, especially focusing on the roles of the neurotrophic factor BDNF and its pathways:

- **Neurotrophic Factor Production**:
  - **Enhanced Secretion of BDNF and Growth Factors**: Physical exercise boosts the production of Brain-Derived Neurotrophic Factor (BDNF) along with other growth factors. The increase in physical activity stimulates the body's metabolic systems, which, in turn, triggers the release of these crucial proteins in the brain.
  - **Activation of Signaling Pathways**: When BDNF binds to its specific receptor, TrkB, located on the surfaces of neurons, it initiates a cascade of signaling events inside the cell. This pathway, primarily through the activation of proteins like PLCγ, PI3K, and ERK, leads to changes in gene expression and protein synthesis essential for neuron function.

- **Neuron Growth and Survival**:
  - **Promotion of Neuron Growth and Survival**: The signaling pathways activated by BDNF enhance the growth and survival of neurons by influencing gene expression that

supports neuronal health and functionality.

- **Processes of Dendritic Branching and Synaptogenesis**: As a direct consequence of enhanced growth signals, neurons extend their dendrites (the branches that receive signals from other neurons) and form more synapses (the points of communication between neurons). This growth and connectivity are crucial for effective neural network functioning.

- **Synaptic Plasticity**:
  - **Modification of Synaptic Plasticity**: Increased levels of BDNF improve synaptic plasticity, which refers to the ability of synapses to strengthen or weaken over time in response to increases or decreases in their activity.
  - **Changes in Synaptic Strength and Structure**: Synaptic modifications include the strengthening of synaptic connections through processes such as the insertion of more receptor proteins into the synaptic membrane, making the synapse more responsive to neurotransmitters.

- **Long-Term Potentiation (LTP)**:
  - **Facilitation of LTP by BDNF**: One of the remarkable effects of exercise-induced BDNF is its role in facilitating Long-Term Potentiation (LTP). LTP is considered one of the major cellular mechanisms that underlies learning and memory. It involves a long-lasting enhancement in signal transmission between two neurons that results from their synchronous stimulation.

This guide articulates how physical activity, by elevating BDNF and related pathways, substantially contributes to the adaptability and efficiency of the brain's neural networks. The enhancement of such biochemical pathways not only supports cognitive functions like learning and memory but also promotes overall brain health, underscoring the profound impact of regular exercise on brain dynamics. Through this clear and structured exposition, the connections between regular physical activities and cognitive health become evident, encouraging a proactive approach to both physical and mental wellness.

Imagine your brain is like a smartphone receiving regular software updates; each new experience or skill you learn prompts your brain to update its functionalities, improving performance and efficiency. This process in your brain is known as neuroplasticity. Just as a software update can enhance a device's features or fix previous bugs, neuroplasticity modifies neural connections to optimize brain function, based on the demands placed upon it.

In the same way that an athlete trains to perfect a technique or increase endurance, your brain strengthens pathways that are frequently used and prunes away the less needed ones. For instance, practicing a new language strengthens the neural circuits involved in language processing and recall, much like a runner strengthens leg muscles.

These day-to-day modifications to our 'mental muscles' and 'brain software' help us adapt to new challenges, learn from past experiences, and recover from traumas. Just as consistent training sharpens an athlete's performance, regular mental exercises like puzzles, learning tasks, or even navigating new routes during your commute, can refine and enhance your brain's ability to respond swiftly and efficiently. This enhancement is vital not just for solving complex problems but for everyday decision-making and emotional regulation, proving that neuroplasticity isn't just a fascinating scientific fact—it's a daily driver of personal growth and adaptation.

The recovery journey of Gabby Giffords, alongside the historical case of Phineas Gage, underscores the profound impacts of neuroplasticity in the context of brain injuries. Gabby Giffords, a U.S. Congresswoman, suffered a severe brain injury due to a gunshot wound in 2011. Her recovery has been a testament to the brain's ability to adapt and reorganize itself following significant trauma. Intensive rehabilitation, encompassing physical, speech, and occupational therapies, leveraged the principles of neuroplasticity to rewire her brain. Over time, different brain regions took over functions that were managed by the damaged areas, enabling her to regain abilities that were initially lost due to the injury.

In contrast, Phineas Gage was a railroad construction foreman who, in 1848, survived an accident wherein a large iron rod was driven completely through his head, damaging much of his brain's left frontal lobe. Remarkably, Gage lived for another 12 years after the incident. His case was one of the first to suggest a link between brain trauma and personality change, providing early evidence that the brain affects social and emotional behaviors. The shift in his behavior and subsequent partial recovery also highlighted the brain's plasticity, showing its capacity to adapt to injuries.

Both cases, although centuries apart, demonstrate the real-life impacts of neuroplasticity. Giffords' recovery, supported by modern medical interventions, and Gage's historical accident provide compelling evidence of how the human brain can undergo significant changes to adapt to new circumstances brought about by injury. These instances not only illustrate eventual adaptability and functional reorganization but also underscore the ongoing advancements in our understanding of neuroplasticity and its potential to aid recovery. Each narrative weaves through the complex tapestry of brain recovery, showcasing resilience and the critical role of targeted rehabilitation in harnessing the brain's adaptive capabilities.

Let's take a deeper look at the intricate neuronal pathways and mechanisms that played pivotal roles in the recovery processes of Gabby Giffords and the neuroplastic changes observed after Phineas Gage's brain injury.

- **Neuronal Pathways and Cell Types Involved**:
Giffords' injury primarily affected her left hemisphere, crucial for language and speech. The brain regions such as Broca's area, responsible for speech production, and surrounding cortical areas, experienced trauma. Remarkably, her brain began to reassign some of these functions to adjacent, less damaged areas and even to counterparts in the right hemisphere. On the other hand, Phineas Gage's injury disrupted frontal lobe functions, which include emotional regulation and decision-making. Subsequent neuroplasticity likely involved compensatory activities by other frontal regions and perhaps the prefrontal cortex, trying to take over some of the lost executive functions.

- **Molecular Mechanisms**:

Post-injury, the role of neurotrophic factors like Brain-Derived Neurotrophic Factor (BDNF) becomes crucial. These proteins support the survival of existing neurons and encourage the growth of new neurons and synapses. In response to physical and cognitive therapy, the expression of BDNF likely surged in both Giffords' and Gage's brains, facilitating recovery. Besides BDNF, other molecular players include neurotransmitters like glutamate and GABA, which help re-establish and modify synaptic connections during recovery.

- **Changes in Synaptic Connections**:

The loss and subsequent formation of synaptic connections are central to understanding neuroplasticity in both cases. For Giffords, therapies aimed at language and motor skills would have stimulated synaptic strengthening and neurogenesis in areas taking over lost functions. Synaptic pruning—where less-used connections are eliminated—also plays a role, helping her brain streamline functions more efficiently in the recovery phase. For Gage, changes in synaptic connections might explain shifts in personality and social behavior, as neurons in undamaged parts of the brain formed new pathways to compensate for the damaged regions.

These insights into the cellular level underline the brain's remarkable ability to adapt following severe injuries. Understanding these processes not only helps in appreciating the scientific complexity of neuroplasticity but also highlights the broader implications for rehabilitation and recovery strategies in neurological injuries. Through such detailed exploration, we gain not only deeper scientific insights but also a greater appreciation for the resilience and adaptability of the human brain.

Imagine your brain as a bustling city, with roads and pathways connecting every corner. Each time you learn a new skill or pick up a new hobby, it's like constructing a new road within this city. Neuroplasticity is the brain's way of building these new routes. Initially, navigating a new route might be challenging, much like the first time you try to bake a cake or solve a crossword puzzle. The process requires attention and effort, with each attempt laying down more pavement, making the route clearer and more familiar.

As you repeat the activity, the connections strengthen, similar to a path becoming well-trodden and easier to travel. This is your brain optimizing the route for more efficient travel in the future. Just as a well-used road is widened and improved over time to accommodate more traffic, the neural pathways associated with your new skills become faster and more efficient the more you use them.

This process isn't just about building new roads but also deciding which old ones might not be necessary anymore, similar to how a city plans its development. Neuroplasticity also involves pruning away the less traveled routes to make space for the most useful ones, ensuring your cognitive resources are allocated effectively. This is why, over time, practiced skills become second nature, and unneeded information fades away—like how you naturally remember the steps to your favorite dance moves but might forget a math formula you haven't used since high school.

Understanding neuroplasticity in this way highlights its role in constantly reshaping our brain's landscape based on our experiences and activities. It showcases the brain's dynamic capacity to adapt and optimize itself, illustrating that, with repeated practice, any challenging skill can become just another well-paved road in the intricate city of our mind.

Here is the breakdown on the molecular mechanisms involved in neuroplasticity during skill acquisition and cognitive pruning, designed to deepen your understanding of how our brains adapt and refine their functions:

- **Synaptic Formation and Strengthening**:
   - **Role of Neurotransmitters**: Neurotransmitters such as glutamate play a pivotal role in synaptic potentiation. When you learn something new, glutamate is released at the synapse, binding to receptors on the post-synaptic neuron which increases the probability of neuron firing, strengthening the synaptic connection.
   - **Calcium Ions and Synaptic Plasticity**: Following the neurotransmitter interaction, calcium ions flow into neurons through channels in the post-synaptic membrane. These ions act as second messengers, triggering a cascade of intracellular events involving protein kinases such as CaMKII and proteins like cAMP response element-binding (CREB). These proteins facilitate changes in gene expression that strengthen the synaptic connection, making the transmission of electrical signals more efficient over time.

- **Neural Circuit Configuration**:
   - **Formation of New Neural Circuits**: When you acquire new skills, the brain doesn't just modify existing neural connections; it also forms new ones. This process involves neurotrophins like Brain-Derived Neurotrophic Factor (BDNF). BDNF fosters the growth of new dendritic spines, sites of synaptic connection, which are essential for forming new neural circuits.
   - **Reinforcement of Neural Circuits**: With repeated use, these new circuits undergo a process called Long-Term Potentiation (LTP), where their synaptic connections become stronger and more efficient. This repetition enhances synaptic efficiency, allowing for quicker and smoother execution of the learned skill.

- **Synaptic Pruning**:
   - **Cellular Processes Leading to Synaptic Degradation**: Synaptic pruning is an essential aspect of neuroplasticity, where less-used synaptic connections are weakened and eventually removed. This process involves microglia, the brain's immune cells, which engulf and digest weak synapses. Proteins in the complement cascade mark these weak synapses for removal, ensuring that microglia target them accurately.
   - **Cognitive Efficiency and Resource Allocation**: By eliminating less-used connections, the brain efficiently reallocates its resources towards more active circuits, improving cognitive efficiency. This ensures that the brain remains adaptable, capable of learning new skills while retaining the most valuable information.

This detailed exploration of the molecular and cellular

mechanisms underpinning neuroplasticity illustrates the brain's remarkable ability to adaptively rewire itself. Understanding these processes not only enhances your appreciation of brain functionality but also underscores the critical role of continuous learning and the application of new skills in maintaining cognitive vitality.

Understanding neuroplasticity not just enlightens us about brain function but also empowers us to take control of our mental fitness. The brain's ability to reshape itself in response to our actions and experiences offers a powerful tool for personal development. By engaging in activities that challenge the intellect, from learning a new language to mastering a musical instrument, we can effectively encourage our brains to grow and adapt. Similarly, regular physical exercise not only benefits the body but also enhances cognitive reserve and resilience due to its positive effects on brain structure.

The implications of this knowledge are profound, suggesting that our daily habits and chosen activities have the potential to strengthen our minds. Just as a gardener nurtures a garden, maintaining and enhancing its beauty and productivity, we can nurture our brains, enhancing their functionality and longevity. This perspective not only changes how we view our capacity for growth but also reinforces the importance of continuous learning and mental engagement as vital components of a healthy lifestyle.

Embracing this understanding means we view brain health as an active, ongoing process. It encourages a proactive approach to mental fitness, emphasizing that our choices can significantly impact our cognitive capabilities and overall well-being. By fostering a lifestyle that values and incorporates brain-enhancing activities, we optimize our potential for maintaining sharp, agile minds well into our later years.

HISTORICAL PERSPECTIVES

The concept of neuroplasticity, the brain's ability to reorganize itself by forming new neural connections, has not always held its current status as a fundamental principle of neuroscience. Initially met with skepticism, the idea that the adult brain can change in response to experience clashed with the long-standing belief in its immutable nature. This chapter of 'Historical Perspectives' details the transformative journey from these early doubts to the eventual acceptance and celebration of neuroplasticity in the scientific community.

Through a series of groundbreaking studies and pivotal shifts in understanding, this once controversial idea has reshaped our approach to brain science, rehabilitation, and education. From the seminal works of researchers like Santiago Ramón y Cajal to modern advancements providing real-time insights into the brain's dynamic capacities, the narrative of neuroplasticity is rich with innovation and discovery. Each milestone not only challenged the prevailing dogmas of their times but also progressively unveiled the adaptable and resilient nature of the human brain.

This chapter aims to unpack these developments with clarity and precision, providing you with a thorough understanding of how the field's evolution impacts both theoretical research and practical applications today. In understanding this history, we gain more than knowledge;

we learn to appreciate the resilience inherent in both the human brain and the scientific pursuit of truth.

In the nascent stages of studying neuroplasticity, the concept encountered significant skepticism. Traditionally, the scientific community held a rigid view that the adult brain was fixed, both in structure and in its functions, with no capacity for change after critical developmental periods in childhood. This belief was so deeply ingrained that early observations suggesting the contrary were often dismissed or overlooked.

The tide began to turn with the meticulous work of pioneering researchers. Santiago Ramón y Cajal, often called the father of modern neuroscience, proposed that connections within the brain were not fixed but could grow stronger or weaker. He suggested that these changes were dependent on the life experiences of the individual, a radical idea at the time.

However, the acceptance of these ideas did not occur overnight. These early hints at neuroplasticity faced rigid opposition rooted in the then-dominant theory of brain immutability. To make this concept relatable: imagine trying to persuade someone that a piece of well-set concrete can flow and change shape. That was the scale of challenge early neuroplasticity theorists faced.

Cajal's theories slowly gained traction as more evidence emerged from various corners of the globe. Experiments showing recovery of function after neurological damage, for instance, could not easily be explained by the old paradigm that the brain's anatomy was unchangeable.

Detailing these early stages helps underscore the sheer tenacity and curiosity driving scientific progress. It also highlights a broader lesson about the importance of questioning established ideas and being open to new evidence, a principle that is as crucial in everyday problem-solving as it is in complex scientific inquiry. In understanding these challenges and how they were overcome, one gains not only insight into the neuroplasticity itself but also an appreciation for the dynamic and ever-evolving nature of scientific understanding.

Let's take a deeper look at the groundbreaking experiments and scientific evidence that cemented the early theories of neuroplasticity, transforming our understanding of the brain's adaptability.

- **Key Experiments**:
Early experiments that profoundly impacted the concept of neuroplasticity include the study of neurogenesis in rodents. Researchers like Joseph Altman used autoradiography to trace the incorporation of thymidine into replicating DNA, demonstrating that new neurons could be created in the adult rat brain. Another landmark study involved mapping the cortical representations in monkeys before and after sensory deprivation or nerve damage to an arm. These studies, led by Michael Merzenich, showed that the brain regions previously associated with the now non-functional limb became responsive to other sensory inputs, proving significant malleability at the neural level.

- **Evidential Breakthroughs**:
A pivotal moment in neuroscience came with the application of functional magnetic resonance imaging (fMRI) to observe changes in brain activity in real-time. This technology provided visual, empirical evidence that learning and experience could alter the functional organization of the brain. The studies conducted by neuroscientists like Helen Neville and Elissa Newport demonstrated how language acquisition in early childhood could shape auditory processing regions specific to language sounds, offering substantial evidence of neuroplasticity in humans.

- **Impact of These Discoveries**:
The discoveries from these experiments presented a radical departure from the previously accepted doctrine that the adult brain was static. This new understanding opened doors for innovative approaches to therapy and rehabilitation. For instance, the concept of constraint-induced movement therapy, which emerged from understanding that activity and use could guide neural reorganization, revolutionized rehabilitation approaches for stroke and injury patients. This therapy involves restricting the use of a healthy limb, thus forcing the use of the impaired one, promoting cortical reorganization and functional improvement.

These meticulous experiments and the ensuing revelations not only underscored the brain's dynamic potential but also profoundly influenced both academic theories and practical applications in medicine and psychology. By grounding these scientific milestones in clear, engaging explanations, this deeper exploration enhances comprehension of how the brave inquiries of past researchers have paved the way for modern advancements in treating and understanding human cognitive and physical capabilities.

The modern understanding of neuroplasticity has been shaped by several key paradigm shifts that overturned the once rigid perception of the brain's ability to change. Initially, the prevailing belief was that the adult brain was largely immutable after critical developmental periods in childhood and adolescence. This notion began to shift notably in the mid-20th century, primarily due to the work of Canadian psychologist Donald Hebb. Hebb introduced the idea that synaptic connections could strengthen through repeated use, encapsulated in what is now known as Hebb's law: "Neurons that fire together, wire together." This concept laid the foundational understanding that experiences can modify the synaptic connections within the brain.

Another significant shift occurred with advancements in neuroimaging technologies, such as MRI and PET scans, which allowed scientists to observe the brain's activity and its changes in real time. These tools provided clear, visual representations of how learning and experiences physically alter brain structure—demonstrating, for example, that taxi drivers navigating complex city streets have greater development in the brain areas associated with spatial memory.

Moreover, the field of neuroplasticity expanded rapidly

with the realization that the adult brain can not only change with experience but also generate new neurons, a process known as neurogenesis. This overturned decades of certainty that the human brain could not produce new neurons after early development. Studies showing how activities like exercise and cognitive engagement stimulate neurogenesis have revolutionized approaches to everything from mental health therapy to cognitive decline in aging.

These paradigm shifts have collectively nurtured a more dynamic view of the brain, emphasizing its adaptability and continuous potential for change. They underscore the importance of lifelong learning and mental activity in maintaining cognitive health and have profoundly influenced therapeutic strategies for brain injuries and neurodegenerative diseases, illustrating that the brain has a remarkable capacity to rewire and heal itself given the right conditions.

Understanding neuroplasticity involves delving into specific key experimental studies, technological strides in neuroimaging, and practical therapeutic applications influenced by these scientific insights.

Key Experimental Studies:
One fundamental study in neuroplasticity was conducted by Paul Bach-y-Rita in the 1960s, who used tactile stimulation devices to help individuals with sensory loss compensate for dysfunction, illustrating that the brain could reorganize sensory functions. Subjects of the study were individuals with disabilities, and the methodology involved tactile visual substitution systems. The main finding was that

subjects could interpret visual information through tactile input, demonstrating the brain's ability to reroute and adapt sensory processing.

Another significant study involved examining stroke patients who had lost motor functions. Researchers applied constraint-induced movement therapy where the unaffected limb was restrained, forcing use of the affected limb. This method allowed them to observe, using functional MRI, how new neural pathways could form to compensate for damaged areas. Results showed improved motor function and a change in cortical representation areas associated with motor skills.

Technological Advances in Neuroimaging:
MRI (Magnetic Resonance Imaging) and PET (Positron Emission Tomography) scans have been instrumental in advancing our understanding of neuroplasticity. MRI uses strong magnetic fields and radio waves to create detailed images of organs and tissues in the body, including the brain. PET scans involve injecting a small amount of radioactive material into the body to reveal how tissues and organs are functioning, highlighting areas of high chemical activity, such as those involved in neuroplastic changes.

These tools have been crucial in studies like those tracking changes in the brain's activity before and after cognitive therapy, or during learning processes, providing visual proof of neuroplasticity. For instance, researchers have used these technologies to show how meditation and structured cognitive exercises can lead to significant changes in brain structure and function over time.

Impact of Discoveries on Therapeutic Approaches:

The discoveries in neuroplasticity have revolutionized therapeutic approaches for conditions previously deemed irreversible. For example, cognitive-behavioral therapy (CBT) and physical rehabilitation strategies now incorporate tasks designed to engage neuroplastic mechanisms. These therapies are structured around activities that promote brain adaptability to improve cognitive and physical functions affected by conditions like stroke, traumatic brain injury, or neurodegenerative diseases.

Applications such as using computerized brain-training software to delay cognitive decline in elderly patients leverage neuroplasticity by keeping cognitive pathways active and engaged. Similarly, motor skill therapies for stroke recovery focus on repeating specific movements to help forge new neural pathways, effectively regaining lost abilities.

Through these examples, it becomes evident how deepened insights into neuroplasticity not only enhance scientific understanding but also practical application in improving human health and recovery processes, showcasing the profound capacity of the brain to adapt and reorganize in response to experience and training.

Advancements in technology have played a pivotal role in deepening our understanding of neuroplasticity, facilitating significant progress both in research and in practical applications. Initially, insights into the brain's adaptability were limited by the available investigative tools, but the introduction of Magnetic Resonance Imaging (MRI) and Positron Emission Tomography (PET) scans revolutionized this field. MRI and PET scans allow researchers to observe the brain's structure and function in real time, offering a window into the dynamic changes occurring within.

For example, MRI technology can track how specific areas of the brain react to various stimuli and how these areas change following injury or cognitive therapy. Such imaging has provided clear evidence that activities like learning a new language or recovering motor skills post-stroke can literally reshape the brain's neural networks. On the other hand, PET scans contribute by tracking metabolic processes in the brain, helping to pinpoint which areas are most active during certain tasks, which furthers our understanding of functional changes associated with neuroplasticity.

These technologies have not just enhanced scientific research but have also dramatically improved clinical outcomes. In the therapeutic context, real-time brain imaging guides more targeted interventions in neurorehabilitation. Therapists can now see how different parts of the brain respond to treatments, allowing them to tailor their approaches to maximize recovery and functional improvements in patients with brain injuries or neurodegenerative diseases.

Furthermore, the development of non-invasive brain stimulation techniques, such as transcranial magnetic stimulation (TMS), offers another layer of intervention that capitalizes on our understanding of neuroplasticity. By targeting specific brain regions, TMS can encourage the formation of neural connections, which can be crucial for patients recovering from strokes or dealing with depression.

Each technological stride not only adds a piece to the neuroplasticity puzzle but also exponentially expands the potential applications of this knowledge, directly impacting the quality of life for many. These tools underscore the dynamic capacity of the brain to adapt and have shifted the paradigm from one of limitation to one of vast potential, reflecting a matured understanding of the brain's complexity and adaptability.

Here is the breakdown on how MRI and PET scans contribute to our understanding of neuroplasticity, providing a detailed view of the technical processes and their implications in observing and understanding brain adaptability:

- **MRI Technology**:
    - **Image Generation**: MRI scans utilize strong magnetic fields and radio waves to create detailed images of the brain. The process involves aligning the nuclear magnetization of hydrogen atoms in water molecules within the brain tissue to produce a detailed image of the brain's internal structures.
    - **Observations of Structural Changes**: After interventions such as cognitive therapy or language learning, MRI scans have shown changes in the gray matter density and white matter pathways. For instance, increases in gray matter in the hippocampus have been observed in individuals engaging in intensive memory training.

- **Correlation with Cognitive Improvements**: These structural changes, observable with MRI scans, correspond with improvements in cognitive abilities. For example, increased cortical thickness in language areas of the brain has been linked to enhanced language proficiency, and similar patterns are seen in recovery phases following brain injuries, indicating functional restoration and compensation.

- **PET Scan Technology**:
  - **Conducting a PET Scan**: A PET scan involves injecting a small amount of radioactive tracer into the bloodstream. This tracer accumulates in the brain areas that are most active, emitting positrons that are detected by the scanner to produce images showing brain activity.
  - **Highlighting Neurological Activity**: During cognitive tasks involving memory or learning, PET scans can highlight increased metabolic activity in specific brain regions like the prefrontal cortex and hippocampus, showcasing areas involved in processing and storing new information.
  - **Contribution to Understanding Neuroplastic Changes**: PET scan findings reveal which brain areas are recruited for new tasks and how their involvement changes with practice or following injury, providing insights into the dynamic process of neuroplastic adaptation.

- **Technological Synergy**:
  - **Comprehensive View of Neuroplasticity**: By combining data from MRI and PET scans, researchers gain a more complete picture of both the structural and functional aspects of neuroplasticity. This integrative approach allows for the correlation of anatomical changes

with shifts in brain activity patterns.

- **<u>Case Study in Neurorehabilitation</u>**: An example of this synergy is seen in stroke rehabilitation studies, where combined MRI and PET data helped tailor therapies based on individual neuroplastic potential, leading to optimized recovery strategies customized to how each patient's brain reorganizes itself post-injury.

Through the detailed understanding of these technologies, it becomes clear how they not only enhance our grasp of neuroplasticity but also directly influence the development of effective therapeutic interventions, tapping into the brain's inherent capacity to reconfigure itself. This understanding underscores the importance of ongoing advancements in neuroimaging as pivotal to both scientific research and clinical practice.

Imagine Paul Bach-y-Rita as an architect who fundamentally redesigned our understanding of what a building—or in his case, the human brain—can do. Just as an architect finds innovative ways to refurbish an old structure to meet new needs, Bach-y-Rita discovered that the brain could rewire itself to restore lost functions through what's known as sensory substitution. For instance, he developed a device that helped individuals who were blind "see" via tactile sensations, essentially repurposing the sense of touch to feed visual information to the brain. This is similar to converting an old warehouse into a high-tech office space, using existing structures in novel ways.

Michael Merzenich, on the other hand, might be likened to a master gardener who understands how to cultivate a plot of land to maximize its yield over different seasons. In the landscape of the brain, Merzenich showed how practicing certain tasks could essentially cultivate stronger, more efficient neural connections, much like how pruning and tending to a garden encourages stronger plant growth. His work illuminated how targeted exercises could rehabilitate areas of the brain affected by injury or age-related decline, very much similar to how a gardener restores a neglected garden to its former glory or even better.

Both these pioneers have shown that the brain, rather than being a static 'building' or an unchangeable 'garden', is capable of remarkable transformations. Whether by rehabilitating an old structure to meet current needs or by nurturing growth to increase resilience, their contributions underscore an essential message: with the right interventions, the brain can adapt to continue functioning optimally, which has profound implications for everything from education to treating brain injuries and beyond. Through their innovative work, we've learned not just the 'how' of brain adaptability but also its 'why'—its crucial role in our capacity to learn, heal, and thrive, reflecting the ongoing dance of structure and flexibility inherent in both nature and human ingenuity.

The evolution of neuroplasticity, from a contentious notion to a pivotal concept in neuroscience, offers a profound view of how our understanding of the brain has transformed over the centuries. This journey through historical milestones not only illustrates the tenacity and foresight of pioneering researchers but also highlights the significant shifts in scientific thinking—shifts that have paved the way for today's innovative neuroscientific research and interventions.

Each milestone, from Santiago Ramón y Cajal's early observations of neuronal changes to the advent of neuroimaging technologies that allow us to see these changes in real time, has contributed to a more dynamic understanding of the brain. We've learned that the brain is not an immutable organ but a plastic one, continuously shaped by experiences and capable of remarkable recovery. This realization has had transformative implications for clinical practices, offering new avenues for rehabilitation and therapy in the face of injuries and neurodegenerative diseases.

Reflecting on these developments, it becomes clear how each breakthrough, each persistent question, and each novel approach has not only enhanced our grasp of human biology but also improved our ability to heal and rehabilitate. As this chapter closes, the legacy of these scientific endeavors encourages us to continue exploring, questioning, and expanding our knowledge, reminding us that in the realm of neuroscience, the potential for discovery—and recovery—is ceaseless.

MECHANISMS OF PLASTICITY

Neuroplasticity stands at the heart of modern neuroscience, challenging old notions and revealing that the brain is not an unchangeable organ bound by the limits of early development. This crucial concept teaches us that the brain can remodel itself continuously through life in response to new knowledge, experiences, and even injuries. It forms a core understanding essential for deciphering how individuals learn, adapt, and recover, showing us that the brain is as dynamic as life itself.

In exploring neuroplasticity, we unravel how synaptic connections between neurons are not static but are fluid, strengthening or weakening based on neuronal activity. This adaptability is not just a minor detail in the story of the human brain; it is a fundamental feature that allows for the recovery from strokes, the relearning of lost skills, and the everyday processing of myriad stimuli gathered through interactions with the world around us.

As we dive deeper into this topic, the discussions aim not just to inform but to transform abstract scientific concepts into clear, relatable knowledge. By understanding neuroplasticity, we gain insights not only into how the brain works but also how we can influence its functioning to enhance our cognitive abilities, rehabilitate injuries, and potentially delay the effects of aging. This chapter sets the stage to explore these mechanisms in detail, providing a window into the ever-adaptive landscape of the human brain without overstating its complexity or journey.

Synaptic plasticity is the brain's ability to strengthen or weaken synaptic connections in response to varying levels of activity, a process underlying learning and memory. Two crucial mechanisms within this process are long-term potentiation (LTP) and long-term depression (LTD), each playing a distinctive role in how experiences and information are encoded within neural circuits.

Long-term potentiation (LTP) can be thought of as the brain's method of turning up the volume on specific neural pathways. It occurs when frequent activation of a particular synapse leads to an increased efficacy in synaptic transmission over time. This is similar to a path in a forest becoming clearer and more navigable the more it is traveled. During LTP, certain receptors on the postsynaptic neuron become more sensitive to neurotransmitters, the brain's chemical messengers, effectively boosting the signal across the synapse.

On the opposite end, long-term depression (LTD) is similar to the brain turning down the volume. This process involves the weakening of synaptic connections that results from a lesser degree or frequency of synaptic activity. It's like a less-traveled forest path gradually becoming overgrown and harder to traverse. LTD helps eliminate old or less useful connections, making way for newer, more relevant pathways.

Both LTP and LTD are vital for the brain's adaptability. They allow the brain to prioritize certain memories and learnings over others, adapting to new information or forgetting what is no longer necessary. These processes ensure that synaptic connections — the points where neurons communicate — remain as efficient as possible, enhancing the brain's ability to react to changes and new challenges efficiently.

Understanding these concepts does more than just provide insight into how memories are made or lost; it unlocks the broader implications of synaptic activity on cognitive functions, brain health, and our overall learning experiences. By grasping the simple yet profound mechanics of LTP and LTD, anyone can appreciate the brain's incredible ability to adapt, learn from, and interact with the world in ever-changing ways.

Let's take a deeper look at the complex molecular mechanisms involved in long-term potentiation (LTP) and long-term depression (LTD), crucial processes enabling synaptic plasticity, which underpins learning and memory.

- **Receptors and Ion Channels**:
  - **Types of Receptors**: In the context of LTP, NMDA (N-methyl-D-aspartate) and AMPA (α-amino-3-hydroxy-5-methyl-4-isoxazolepropionic acid) receptors play pivotal roles. NMDA receptors act as molecular coincidence detectors, requiring both ligand binding and a pre-existing depolarization of the neuron to activate. AMPA receptors, on the other hand, primarily respond to glutamate and are more readily activated without the need for pre-

depolarization.

- **Calcium Dynamics**: Activation of NMDA receptors during LTP leads to an influx of calcium ions into the neuron. These ions act as a crucial secondary messenger within the cell, triggering various signaling cascades that affect ion channels and other cellular mechanisms.

- **Biochemical Pathways**:
- **Calcium/Calmodulin-Dependent Protein Kinase II (CaMKII)**: This enzyme plays a critical role in LTP. Activated by the increased intracellular calcium, CaMKII phosphorylates various proteins, including AMPA receptors, enhancing their conductance and increasing the synaptic response to glutamate.
- **Transcription and Translation Changes**: Following the activation of pathways like CaMKII, changes occur in the nucleus of the neuron where specific genes are upregulated or downregulated, leading to the production of proteins that consolidate long-lasting synaptic changes. This enhancement or reduction in protein synthesis is critical for strengthening or weakening synapses, respectively.

- **Synaptic Changes**:
- **Structural Modifications**: LTP often results in the growth of new dendritic spines, which provide additional postsynaptic surface area for more synaptic connections. In contrast, LTD can lead to the shrinkage or pruning of spines, effectively decreasing the complexity and connectivity of neurons.
- **Functional Implications**: These structural changes physically manifest the strengthening or weakening of synaptic efficacy, aligning with the cognitive processes such

as learning (LTP) or forgetting (LTD).

This more detailed examination sheds light on how a cascade of molecular and cellular events triggered by experiences and learning exercises translates into the physical restructuring and functional re-tuning of the brain's neural circuitry. Understanding these intricate processes not only fascinates scientifically but also offers insight into potential therapeutic approaches for enhancing cognitive function or ameliorating neurological conditions. Through a clear understanding of these mechanisms, we begin to see the profound capability of the brain to adapt and remodel itself continually—a feature central to our interactions with, and adaptations to, our ever-changing environment.

The cellular mechanisms underlying neuroplasticity are as fundamental as they are fascinating, acting as the core processes through which the brain alters its structure to accommodate new learning and memory consolidation. At the heart of these processes is the ability of neurons to form, strengthen, weaken, or eliminate their connecting points, known as synapses, in response to various stimuli.

Firstly, the formation of new synaptic connections, or synaptogenesis, is facilitated by the release of specific proteins and growth factors in the brain. These substances promote the sprouting of dendrites (the receiving part of a neuron) and axons (the transmitting part), encouraging them to reach out and establish new contacts with neighboring neurons. This is similar to laying down new roads in a city to improve connectivity and traffic flow.

Maintaining these connections involves a process called synaptic strengthening, where the efficiency of synaptic transmission is increased. This usually occurs through the mechanism of long-term potentiation (LTP), where repeated stimulation of a particular synapse increases the post-synaptic neuron's sensitivity to its neurotransmitter, much like strengthening a muscle through exercise. This enhances synaptic efficacy and ensures that the pathway remains active and robust.

Conversely, the elimination of synaptic connections, known as synaptic pruning, is equally important. This process removes less-used or weak synapses, a bit like how a gardener prunes dead branches to allow a tree to thrive. Synaptic pruning is crucial during early development and plays a significant role in refining neural circuits according to experiential demands – it helps the brain 'let go' of unnecessary connections to make way for more relevant and efficient pathways.

These dynamic changes in synaptic connections are underpinned by complex biochemical pathways that involve a multitude of enzymes, receptor molecules, and intracellular signaling cascades. They work in concert to transduce the signals necessary for the modulation of synaptic strength in accordance with neuronal activity.

Understanding these intricate cellular mechanisms enriches our appreciation of how the brain learns and adapts. It is not just about forming new connections; it is about selectively strengthening useful connections and eliminating those that are not needed, thereby optimizing brain functions for efficient processing. This dynamic modification process underscores the incredible adaptability of the brain, highlighting its capacity to reorganize itself continually in response to new information or environmental changes. Such knowledge is not only foundational for academic purposes but also offers hopeful avenues for interventions in learning disabilities, psychiatric disorders, and recovery from brain injuries.

Synaptic strengthening and pruning are pivotal in shaping the brain's ability to adapt and learn. Understanding the biochemical pathways and molecular interactions involved provides a fundamental insight into how memories are formed and adjusted.

Beginning with synaptic strengthening, a critical event is the influx of calcium ions through NMDA receptors, which are typically activated when both glutamate binds to them and the postsynaptic neuron is sufficiently depolarized. Once these calcium ions enter the neuron, they trigger a cascade of signals that ultimately lead to changes in gene expression and protein synthesis. These changes increase the density of AMPA receptors at the synaptic site, enhancing synaptic efficacy and thereby strengthening the synaptic connection.

For instance, the activation of calcium/calmodulin-dependent protein kinase II (CaMKII) by calcium ions is one such signaling event. CaMKII phosphorylates AMPA receptors, increasing their activity. It also modifies other proteins within the spine, encouraging structural changes that make the synapse stronger. This process can be thought of as upgrading the hardware in a computer to handle more complex tasks faster and more efficiently.

Turning to the role of glutamate transporters, these are essential in maintaining synaptic efficacy by regulating levels of glutamate, the primary excitatory neurotransmitter in the brain. They help terminate the glutamate signal in synaptic transmission by quickly clearing glutamate from the synaptic cleft, which prevents ongoing activation of receptors and ensures that communication between neurons is crisp and not blurred by residual neurotransmitter.

In synaptic pruning, microglia play a crucial role in identifying and removing less active or weak synapses. This is somewhat similar to pruning in gardening where non-productive or dead branches are cut away to improve the health and productivity of the plant. Microglia digest these unnecessary synaptic elements, facilitating the brain's ability to redirect resources towards strengthening more active and essential synapses. This process enhances the efficiency of neural networks, ensuring that they are tailored to the demands of the environment and the organism's behavioral needs.

This detailed breakdown of the pathways and processes involved in synaptic strengthening and pruning shows how intricately the brain works to adapt and optimize itself. Each molecular interaction and pathway not only plays a role in immediate synaptic changes but also contributes broadly to the cognitive capacities of learning and memory. By understanding these processes, we gain insight into the dynamic and highly adaptable nature of the brain, highlighting its incredible ability to rewire and refine its functions continually.

Just as a gardener nurtures a garden, adjusting to the whims of weather and seasons, so too do environmental factors shape the ever-adaptive terrain of our brains, sculpting the neural pathways through an intricate dance of neuroplasticity. Imagine the brain as a garden — not a static one, but a dynamic ecosystem where each new experience plants a seed, each learned skill waters it, and repetitive practices fertilize the soil, encouraging robust growth.

In this living garden, sunlight and rain are similar to the stimuli we encounter in our daily lives. Just as a plant's growth is influenced by the quality and quantity of light and moisture it receives, our brain's development and adaptive capabilities are profoundly shaped by the variety and intensity of environmental stimuli. A rich, stimulating environment, full of novel experiences and challenges, acts like a nourishing climate, enabling the brain to flourish and expand its neural connections much like flourishing foliage in ideal growing conditions.

Conversely, a lack of sensory stimulation is like a drought to the brain's garden; it hampers the growth of new neural connections, much as parched soil might stunt a seedling's growth. Similarly, if the sculptor — representing our active engagement with the environment — neglects the clay, the sculpture loses its potential form, just as our cognitive abilities might wane without mental exercise and new experiences.

Such analogies not only simplify the complexities of neuroplasticity but also highlight its significance: the brain, like a garden or a piece of art, requires consistent cultivation and creative engagement to reach its full potential. By embracing diverse experiences and continually challenging ourselves, we can ensure that our brain's garden blooms splendidly, vibrant with the lush foliage of enriched neural pathways and vibrant cognitive functions.

Here is the breakdown on the specific neural mechanisms affected by environmental stimuli, providing a deeper insight into how these factors contribute to neuroplasticity:

- **Synaptic Strength**:
  - **Neurotransmitter Role**: Environmental stimuli can alter the release of neurotransmitters such as glutamate and dopamine, which are critical for synaptic transmission. For example, engaging learning activities increase glutamate release, enhancing synaptic efficacy.
  - **Plasticity Markers**: Proteins like Brain-Derived Neurotrophic Factor (BDNF) are upregulated by stimulating environments, leading to enhanced synaptic plasticity. BDNF helps facilitate long-term potentiation (LTP), a process that strengthens synapses.

- **Neural Circuit Formation**:
  - **Neurogenesis**: Continuous learning and sensory stimulation can lead to the generation of new neurons in certain areas of the brain, such as the hippocampus, which

are crucial for memory and learning.

- **Synaptic Pruning**: Effective and repeated use of neural pathways leads to the strengthening of these pathways while rarely used synapses are pruned away, making neural circuits more efficient. This process is guided by signals from neuronal activity that dictate which connections are reinforced and which are eliminated.

- **Molecular Cascade**:
- **Activation of Receptors**: Environmental challenges trigger receptors like NMDA and AMPA, which play vital roles in synaptic plasticity. Activation of NMDA receptors, for example, allows calcium ions to enter neurons, setting off a series of intracellular reactions.
- **Signaling Pathways**: Calcium influx activates signaling molecules such as CaMKII and CREB. These molecules initiate further signaling cascades that ultimately lead to changes in gene expression, influencing synaptic strength and circuit architecture.
- **Protein Synthesis**: The molecular signals eventually lead to the synthesis of new proteins that are essential for reinforcing the structural changes in synapses necessary for adaptive behavior.

This comprehensive exploration from neurotransmitters to protein synthesis illustrates how environmental stimuli intricately influence neural mechanisms, shaping the brain's ability to adapt through neuroplasticity. Understanding these connections deepens one's appreciation of how everyday interactions with our surroundings have a profound impact on our cognitive functions, ultimately influencing who we are and how we interact with the world. By delving into these scientific aspects, one gains a practical understanding that connects these phenomena to everyday experiences, bringing the dynamic world of brain science closer to general comprehension.

Recent technological advances in neuroimaging and molecular biology have significantly enhanced our understanding of neuroplasticity, revealing intricate details of how the brain adapts through life. Functional Magnetic Resonance Imaging (fMRI) and Positron Emission Tomography (PET) scans are at the forefront of these technologies, enabling scientists to visualize brain activity in real time. These imaging techniques can show how different areas of the brain activate during various tasks, allowing researchers to map changes and connections as they occur, much like a traffic controller monitoring the flow of vehicles on multiple roadways.

Simultaneously, advancements in molecular biology have equipped us with sophisticated tools like CRISPR and single-cell RNA sequencing. These tools help identify the roles of specific genes and proteins in brain plasticity, providing a layer-by-layer understanding of the molecular underpinnings. For instance, single-cell RNA sequencing offers insights into the gene expression profiles of individual neurons, helping to distinguish how diverse cellular environments influence neuronal behavior and connectivity.

Such detailed imaging combined with molecular analysis has practical implications in both clinical and educational settings. In medicine, this knowledge is pivotal for developing targeted therapies for neurological disorders, such as bespoke interventions for stroke recovery or cognitive rehabilitation strategies for dementia. In educational spheres, understanding the variables that enhance brain plasticity can inform teaching methods and learning environments that adapt to the unique neural wiring of each student, promoting optimal educational outcomes.

As we continue exploring these technological frontiers, the potential to not only understand but also influence brain plasticity grows. However, it is crucial to approach these advancements with a balanced perspective, acknowledging their limitations—such as the high costs of neuroimaging and the ethical considerations in gene manipulation. Emphasizing responsible usage and continuous innovation, these technologies promise to unlock further secrets of neuroplasticity, potentially revolutionizing our approach to health, education, and beyond. This journey into the brain's adaptability not only furthers scientific inquiry but also serves as a testament to human ingenuity in its quest to decode the most complex organ in the body.

Let's take a deeper look at the advanced technologies of Functional Magnetic Resonance Imaging (fMRI) and Positron Emission Tomography (PET) scans, along with CRISPR and single-cell RNA sequencing, and their instrumental roles in exploring and influencing neuroplasticity.

- **fMRI and PET Scans**:
  - **Process**: fMRI measures brain activity by detecting changes associated with blood flow. When an area of the brain is more active, it consumes more oxygen, and fMRI can detect these areas because oxygenated and deoxygenated

blood have different magnetic properties. PET scans, on the other hand, use a radioactive tracer injected into the bloodstream that accumulates in brain areas with high chemical activity, allowing the detection of metabolic processes and neural activity.

- **Interpreting Changes**: These scanning technologies can track how brain activity patterns change during various cognitive tasks or in response to different environmental stimuli. The ability of fMRI and PET scans to observe these changes over time provides critical insights into the brain's plastic nature, illustrating how experiences rewire neural pathways and affect overall brain function.

- **CRISPR in Neuroplasticity**:
    - **Gene Editing**: CRISPR (Clustered Regularly Interspaced Short Palindromic Repeats) technology allows scientists to edit or modify the DNA of living organisms with precision. In neuroplasticity studies, CRISPR can target and modify genes that are crucial for synaptic development and plastic changes in the brain.
    - **Experimental Applications**: For instance, researchers have used CRISPR to manipulate genes that encode neurotransmitter receptors to observe how changes in these receptors affect learning and memory in animal models. This manipulation helps in understanding how synaptic connections are formed, strengthened, or weakened, directly influencing neuroplasticity.

- **Single-cell RNA Sequencing**:
    - **Isolating Neurons**: This process begins with the isolation of single neurons from a brain sample. Each neuron is separated and encased in a tiny droplet containing

chemicals that burst the cell open, releasing its RNA.

- **Sequencing Methodology**: The extracted RNA is then converted into complementary DNA (cDNA). The cDNA is sequenced, and computational tools are used to analyze the sequences to identify the RNA molecules present in each cell.

- **Insights into Neuroplasticity**: By determining the RNA profiles of individual neurons, scientists can understand how specific genes are expressed in different types of neurons under various conditions. This detailed data allows researchers to trace the pathways of neuroplastic changes, showing how individual cells adapt to learning or environmental challenges.

Through these detailed examinations of fMRI, PET scans, CRISPR, and single-cell RNA sequencing, we gain a robust understanding of the dynamic interactions and modifications occurring within the brain. Each technology not only provides a window into the microscopic workings of neural pathways but also offers tools to potentially guide and enhance cognitive functions through targeted interventions. This union of technology and biology is shaping an exciting era of neuroscience, where deciphering and harnessing the brain's adaptability can lead to substantial advances in both health and education.

Neuroplasticity has captivated the scientific community, thanks largely to remarkable contributions from key researchers who have shaped our understanding of the brain's adaptive capabilities. Donald Hebb, often dubbed the father of neuropsychology, introduced the concept that neurons that fire together wire together, laying the groundwork for understanding how habits and learning patterns influence brain connections. His theoretical models form the backbone of countless strategies in rehabilitative and cognitive therapies today.

On the experimental front, the late Paul Bach-y-Rita was a pioneer in applying neuroplastic principles to real-world therapies. He innovatively used "sensory substitution" devices to aid people with disabilities, showing that the brain could adapt to new sensory inputs in remarkable ways, thus broadening our appreciation for the brain's flexibility.

Eric Kandel's work further solidified the biological basis of neuroplasticity. His research on synaptic changes in the sea slug Aplysia earned him a Nobel Prize and proved that synapses are altered by activity, a phenomenon observable across species, including humans. This finding has profound implications for educational practices and therapies aimed at cognitive enhancement.

Michael Merzenich, another luminary, focused on applied neuroplasticity, pioneering techniques like brain training exercises that have been instrumental in treating learning disabilities and brain injuries. His work underscores the practical impact of neuroplastic research, demonstrating that targeted exercises can rewire the brain, enhancing its functionality.

Together, these researchers have not only advanced the theoretical and practical aspects of neuroplasticity but have also offered hope and solutions to those once considered beyond help by traditional methods. Their legacy continues to inspire innovations in how we might harness the brain's malleability for therapeutic and educational betterment, making their contributions as relevant today as ever.

Neuroplasticity, the brain's remarkable ability to reorganize itself by forming new neural connections throughout life, stands as a central theme in the ever-evolving landscape of neuroscience. This chapter has meticulously unraveled the layers of neuroplasticity, illustrating not only how it occurs but also its significant implications for medicine, education, and our broader understanding of human cognition.

Through advancements in technology and insights from pioneering researchers, we've seen firsthand that the brain is not as rigidly hardwired as once thought. Instead, it is a dynamic entity, continually adapting to new experiences, learning, and even injuries. This adaptability underscores the importance of neuroplasticity in therapeutic strategies, offering new avenues for rehabilitation practices that can aid recovery from neurological disorders, enhance cognitive abilities, and improve the quality of life.

Moreover, grasping the nuances of how environmental factors, lifestyle choices, and structured learning activities can influence brain plasticity empowers individuals to actively enhance their cognitive functions. The roles of technologies like fMRI, PET scans, and molecular biology tools such as CRISPR and single-cell RNA sequencing have been pivotal, offering deeper insights and practical tools for manipulating the pathways that govern neuroplasticity.

In conclusion, neuroplasticity is not merely a scientific concept confined to academic discussions; it is a profound reality that impacts everything from how we recover from brain injuries to how we can optimize mental functioning across the lifespan. As we continue to uncover the mysteries of the brain's plastic nature, we hold in our hands the potential to revolutionize approaches to health, education, and understanding the essence of human intelligence and behavior. This ongoing journey not only propels scientific inquiry but also promises to enhance the human experience in meaningful ways.

PLASTICITY IN LEARNING AND MEMORY

This fundamental process within neuroplasticity is similar to the brain rewiring its own circuitry in response to new experiences, challenges, or environmental changes. By forging new neural pathways or strengthening existing ones, neuroplasticity plays a critical role in our capacity to acquire new skills, store memories, and adapt to novel situations.

Understanding neuroplasticity not only deepens our grasp of cognitive development but also illuminates pathways for enhancing educational methods and therapeutic techniques. It presents a compelling narrative of a brain not fixed in its capacities but continually evolving. This dynamic view encourages a perspective of lifelong learning and adaptability, reinforcing the notion that with the right stimuli or interventions, cognitive enhancement remains within reach at any age.

Thus, as we explore the intricate dance of neurons involved in shaping the human mind, we unveil potent strategies that can significantly influence how effectively we learn, remember, and adapt. Neuroplasticity is not just a subject of academic intrigue; it is a pivotal concept with profound implications for practical applications in educational psychology and beyond, offering promising avenues for future research and implementation.

Neuroplasticity is underpinned by biological processes

that enable the brain to modify its functioning and structure in response to new experiences. Central to these processes are synaptic adjustments—tiny changes at the junctions between neurons that transmit nerve signals. These synaptic adjustments are chiefly responsible for the brain's capacity to learn new information and enhance memory.

Synaptic plasticity, the ability of synapses to strengthen or weaken over time, relies significantly on activity in the neural circuitry. When a neuron frequently sends a signal across the synapse to another neuron, the connection between them strengthens. This phenomenon, known as long-term potentiation (LTP), is like carving a deeper path in a well-trodden trail, making the passage of information more efficient. Conversely, when a synapse is rarely used, it undergoes long-term depression (LTD), weakening the connection much like a seldom-used trail becomes overgrown and hard to navigate.

These mechanisms are pivotal in learning and memory. For example, when learning a new skill, such as playing a piano, repeated practice strengthens the relevant synaptic pathways, making it easier and more automatic to perform over time. This is similar to walking the same path every day until it becomes a clear and easy route.

Understanding these synaptic mechanisms offers invaluable insights into educational strategies that could enhance learning. By targeting these synaptic changes through specific learning activities tailored to strengthen beneficial neural connections, educational methodologies can potentially be optimized to foster better learning outcomes.

The implications of neuroplasticity extend beyond mere academic interest. Insights into how synaptic adjustments can be manipulated have significant repercussions for treating brain injuries and neurodegenerative diseases, where enhancing synaptic plasticity could help regain lost functions or slow disease progression. Thus, a deep appreciation of these biological underpinnings not only elevates one's understanding of the human brain's capabilities but also opens up new avenues for impactful applications in medicine and education, stressing the importance of ongoing research and innovation in this dynamic field.

Let's take a deeper look at the intricate cellular and molecular processes underlying Long-Term Potentiation (LTP) and Long-Term Depression (LTD), crucial phenomena at the heart of synaptic plasticity.

Long-Term Potentiation (LTP):
1. **Neuronal Activity and Neurotransmitter Release**: It begins when a pre-synaptic neuron fires action potentials more frequently, leading to the enhanced release of neurotransmitters like glutamate into the synaptic cleft.

2. **Receptor Activation**: These neurotransmitters bind to post-synaptic receptors such as NMDA (N-methyl-D-aspartate) and AMPA (α-amino-3-hydroxy-5-methyl-4-isoxazolepropionic acid) receptors. While AMPA receptors quickly respond by allowing positively charged ions like sodium to flow into the neuron, creating a postsynaptic potential, NMDA receptors play a pivotal role once they

become active under certain conditions: sufficient neurotransmitter binding and a pre-existing depolarization of the post-synaptic membrane.

3. **Calcium Influx and Signaling Cascades**: Activation of NMDA receptors leads to an influx of calcium ions, which are critical for the next steps. Calcium ions act as a secondary messenger, initiating several signaling pathways inside the neuron, including the activation of enzymes like calmodulin-dependent kinase II (CaMKII) and the cyclic AMP-responsive element-binding protein (CREB).

4. **Gene Transcription and Protein Synthesis**: These enzymes can travel to the nucleus and influence gene expression, leading to the synthesis of new proteins that not only strengthen the existing synaptic connections but also aid in forming new ones.

5. **Synaptic Changes**: The result is a strengthened synapse, with more AMPA receptors inserted into the synaptic membrane and a structurally larger synaptic junction. This enhanced synaptic configuration improves the efficiency of synaptic transmission, locking in the potentiated state.

Long-Term Depression (LTD):

1. **Reduced Neuronal Activity**: Here, the converse occurs. A lower frequency of action potentials leads to reduced release of neurotransmitters.

2. **Receptor Modification and Internalization**: Prolonged low levels of calcium influx through NMDA receptors trigger different signaling cascades that lead to the removal of AMPA receptors from the synaptic membrane.

3. **Decrement in Synaptic Strength**: This receptor internalization reduces the synapse's responsiveness to neurotransmitters, effectively weakening the synaptic

connection.

Understanding these processes in detail is not just academic; knowing how synaptic strength can be modulated provides crucial insights for developing targeted interventions. In education, techniques such as spaced repetition and active recall can be designed to exploit LTP mechanisms, enhancing learning and memory retention. Therapeutically, strategies to modulate these pathways can aid in recovery from neurological disorders, offering hope for conditions from stroke to Alzheimer's disease, where synaptic connections have been damaged or lost.

By demystifying these complex processes, we equip educators, clinicians, and researchers with the knowledge to harness the brain's own mechanisms of change, paving the way for interventions that closely align with our natural neural tendencies and capacities. This understanding embodies a significant stride in linking neuroscience with practical applications, promising a future where education and therapy are deeply informed by our understanding of the brain's innate adaptability.

Imagine you're in a garden, tending to various plants, each requiring different amounts of sunlight, water, and care to thrive. Similarly, educational institutions and therapeutic settings apply the principles of neuroplasticity to cultivate a student's or patient's cognitive abilities, each according to their unique needs and conditions. Just as a gardener uses specific techniques to nurture growth, educators and therapists tailor cognitive exercises and learning strategies to enhance brain functionality.

In school settings, this might look like implementing classroom activities designed to strengthen neural pathways through repetition and challenge, similar to how pruning helps a plant grow healthier by cutting off less necessary parts to redirect resources to flourish blooms. Techniques such as spaced repetition in studying — think of it like watering a plant intermittently but with the right amount to make it absorb nutrients better — help students commit information to long-term memory more efficiently.

In therapy, especially cognitive rehabilitation after a brain injury, the approach is like rehabilitating a garden after a storm. Therapists work to re-establish and sometimes reroute neural pathways, using exercises that promote the brain's ability to form new connections, much like planting new seeds in damaged areas of the garden to bring it back to life.

Understanding neuroplasticity allows educators and therapists to adapt and apply these strategies effectively, ensuring that like a well-maintained garden, each mind they help cultivate can reach its fullest potential. Each approach, tailored to the individual's specific cognitive landscape, works on the underlying neural circuitry, encouraging growth and adaptation in areas most needed. This engagement not only facilitates learning and recovery but also empowers individuals to navigate and interact with the world in enriched, meaningful ways.

Here is the detailed breakdown of the specific neural exercises used in educational and therapeutic settings to enhance neuroplasticity, illustrating their scientific foundation and effectiveness in cognitive development and recovery:

- **Types of Neural Exercises**:
  - **Problem-solving tasks**: These include mathematical problems, logic puzzles, and strategic games which challenge the brain to find solutions and make decisions.
  - **Memory games**: Activities like matching pairs, recalling lists, or sequence games that help strengthen memory recall and retention.
  - **Sensorimotor activities**: These involve coordinated movement and sensory input, such as juggling, playing musical instruments, or interactive video games that require physical interaction.

- **Biological Impact on Neural Pathways**:
  - **Synaptic Plasticity Stimulation**:
    - **Dopamine and Glutamate Role**: These neurotransmitters play crucial roles in reinforcing synaptic connections. Dopamine is linked with reward-learning, enhancing brain circuits that are successfully used in problem-solving. Glutamate acts at synaptic sites to potentiate connections, crucial for memory formation.
    - **Synaptic Strengthening and Weakening**: Activities like problem-solving and memory games increase synaptic strength (through mechanisms like Long-Term Potentiation) as the brain encodes new information. Conversely, disuse of certain neural pathways can lead to synaptic weakening (via Long-Term Depression), streamlining brain function by pruning less-used connections.

- **Practical Applications**:

- **Educational Strategies**:
  - **Customized Learning Approaches**: Techniques such as spaced repetition are used to enhance retention in students, adapting learning sessions based on individual pace and performance.
  - **Interactive Lessons**: Incorporating sensorimotor learning activities in classrooms to engage multiple brain regions simultaneously, promoting more robust neural networks.
- **Cognitive Rehabilitation Therapies**:
  - **Recovery from Neurological Conditions**: Post-stroke or injury, tailored sensorimotor tasks help remodel brain circuits, aiding in regaining lost functionalities.
  - **Adaptability to Individual Needs**: Therapy programs are personalized based on specific deficits or recovery paths, focusing on gradually rebuilding neural strength and flexibility.

This comprehensive exploration of neural exercises and their biological impacts underpins the guidelines for strategically employing neuroplasticity in learning and therapeutic settings. Each method is not just rooted in deep scientific mechanisms but also configured for practical applicability, ensuring that interventions are both scientifically sound and uniquely effective. This understanding lends itself to more informed approaches in both educational frameworks and clinical recovery models, ultimately enhancing cognitive resilience and adaptive learning capacities.

Leveraging neuroplasticity, particularly in educational and therapeutic settings, presents unique challenges due to individual variations in how plasticity manifests. Unlike machines with uniform responses, each human brain reacts differently to similar stimuli, making standardized approaches less effective. These variations can significantly impact the efficacy of strategies designed to enhance learning and memory.

Firstly, the age of an individual plays a crucial role. Younger brains generally exhibit a higher degree of plasticity, making them more adaptable and responsive to neuroplastic interventions compared to older adults. The implication here is that learning strategies that work effectively for children and adolescents might not hold the same potency for adults, whose neural pathways tend to be more established.

Moreover, genetic factors contribute to differences in neuroplastic capabilities. Certain genetic profiles can enhance or impair the neural capacity for adaptation, affecting how well an individual might respond to cognitive training or rehabilitation therapies designed to exploit neuroplasticity. For instance, variations in the production of brain-derived neurotrophic factor (BDNF), a protein that supports neuron growth and connectivity, can influence synaptic plasticity, thereby shaping an individual's learning curve and memory retention.

Additionally, lifestyle factors such as nutrition, exercise, and sleep quality deeply affect neuroplasticity. Poor dietary habits or insufficient physical activity can dampen the neurochemical processes vital for synaptic growth and reorganization, thus stifling the brain's adaptive potential. This requires that any neuroplastic-centered approach in education or therapy also considers the broader lifestyle context of the individual.

The challenge extends to developing personalized methods that not only acknowledge but harness these individual differences. In an educational setting, this might mean adaptive learning technologies that tailor educational content and pace according to a student's specific neural responsiveness, thereby optimizing the learning process. In therapy, it involves creating bespoke rehabilitation programs that align with the patient's unique neuroplastic profile, accounting for their age, genetic predispositions, and lifestyle.

Ultimately, recognizing and addressing the multifaceted layers of individual variations in neuroplasticity is pivotal. Not only does it promise more targeted and effective interventions, but it also heightens our understanding of the brain's complex nature, inviting a more nuanced appreciation of the capabilities and challenges inherent in harnessing its plasticity. Emphasizing these aspects not only educates but also empowers individuals, equipping them with knowledge that significantly impacts real-world applications in learning and health.

Developing personalized educational and therapeutic programs tailored to individual neuroplastic profiles involves a detailed and systematic process. This approach acknowledges the unique neural adaptability of each person, heavily influenced by their genetic makeup, age, lifestyle, and health conditions. Here's a step-by-step guide on how to assess neuroplastic responsiveness and customize interventions accordingly:

Step 1: Initial Assessment
- **Screening for Baseline Neurologic Function**: A series of psychological and cognitive tests are administered to evaluate basic neural functioning and existing cognitive capabilities. Tools may include neuropsychological tests that assess memory, attention, problem-solving, and motor skills.
- **Biomedical Evaluation**: Blood tests, genetic profiling, and brain imaging techniques (like fMRI or PET scans) are used to detect physiological and biochemical indicators, such as levels of brain-derived neurotrophic factor (BDNF), that give insight into an individual's neuroplastic capacity.

Step 2: Profiling Neuroplastic Potential
- **Synaptic Plasticity Measurement**: Advanced neuroimaging and electrophysiological techniques measure how effectively synapses in the brain can strengthen or weaken in response to new stimuli or learning.
- **Cognitive Adaptability Evaluation**: This involves assessing how flexibly the individual can adjust to new learning strategies or environments, critical for tailoring educational and therapeutic approaches.

Step 3: Program Design and Customization
- **Educational and Therapeutic Strategy Design**: Based on the detailed profile created from initial assessments, educational specialists and therapists design a set of personalized learning activities or therapeutic exercises. These are targeted to maximally stimulate neuroplasticity in effective and sustainable ways, considering

factors such as age-related neuroplasticity decline or enhancements specific to the individual's genetic predispositions.

- **Intervention Customization**: Adjustments are continuously made based on ongoing evaluations of the individual's progress. For younger individuals or those with high neuroplastic potential, more aggressive and varied strategies might be employed. In contrast, for older adults or those with restricted neuroplastic capabilities, a more gradual and repetitive approach might be more effective.

Step 4: Interdisciplinary Collaboration

- **Team Coordination**: Neuropsychologists, cognitive neuroscientists, educational specialists, and rehabilitation therapists work as an integrated team. Each professional brings a nuanced understanding of how different facets of neuroplasticity can be optimized for learning and recovery.

- **Continuous Monitoring and Adjustment**: The team regularly reviews the progress of the individual, recalibrating the learning modules or therapy routines to ensure they remain aligned with the evolving neuroplastic capabilities and learning outcomes of the person.

Step 5: Long-term Follow-up and Support

- **Sustained Evaluation and Support**: Long-term support systems and periodic assessments ensure that the benefits of the personalized programs are maintained. Adjustments are made as necessary to accommodate any changes in lifestyle, health status, or personal goals that might affect neuroplasticity.

This comprehensive approach not only maximizes educational outcomes and therapeutic efficacy but also empowers individuals by providing them with tailored strategies that respect and utilize their unique neural wiring. This fosters an environment where learning and recovery are not just possible but are done in alignment with the natural capacities and potential of the brain.

Neuroplasticity has been at the forefront of neuroscience for several decades, with key innovations and research milestones that have profoundly shaped our understanding of learning and therapeutic practices today. One pivotal development was the introduction of the term "neuroplasticity" itself by Polish neuroscientist Jerzy Konorski in 1948, which laid the groundwork for conceptualizing the brain's ability to change structurally and functionally in response to internal and external influences.

A significant breakthrough in this field came from the work of Donald Hebb in 1949, who proposed Hebbian theory. This principle, often summarized as "cells that fire together, wire together," explains how pathways in the brain are strengthened through repeated use, and it has become foundational in understanding how habits and learning form at the neural level. This concept has been applied practically in creating more effective educational strategies and cognitive therapies that align with natural learning patterns.

Another milestone was the experimental demonstration in the late 20th century that the adult brain can generate new neurons, a process called neurogenesis. This overturned the long-held belief that the adult brain was fixed and incapable of such regeneration. Research by scientists like Fred Gage has shown that neurogenesis occurs in areas critical to memory and learning, such as the hippocampus. This discovery has inspired interventions that stimulate brain activity through exercise, cognitive tasks, and even pharmacological agents to enhance mental capabilities and treat neurodegenerative diseases.

In recent years, the advent of sophisticated imaging techniques such as functional magnetic resonance imaging (fMRI) has allowed scientists to observe and measure neuroplastic changes in vivo. This technology offers insights into how specific brain areas activate in real time during various tasks, providing a powerful tool for both researching brain function and developing targeted neuropsychological interventions.

These milestones in neuroplasticity research have not only expanded our theoretical knowledge but also brought tangible benefits to education and therapy. They underline a shift towards more personalized learning experiences and therapeutic approaches that respect each individual's unique neural architecture, optimizing strategies to support cognitive enhancement and rehabilitation. By continually integrating these insights, practitioners and educators can foster environments that substantially improve learning outcomes and patient recovery processes.

The future of neuroplasticity research holds exciting prospects that could transform how we approach learning and cognitive enhancement. As we dive deeper into the brain's ability to rewire itself, emerging technologies and deeper neuroscientific insight promise to revolutionize educational strategies and therapeutic interventions.

One potential advancement lies in the development of more sophisticated neuroimaging techniques. Current methods like fMRI have been instrumental in mapping brain activity, but future improvements might offer higher resolution and real-time tracking of neural pathways as they form, dissolve, or strengthen in response to learning activities or cognitive therapies. This could lead to highly personalized learning regimes, where educational content and the pacing of material are continuously adapted based on direct feedback from an individual's brain activity.

Additionally, genetic research might soon allow us to identify specific genes that influence neuroplasticity, offering revolutionary approaches in personalized education and therapy. Imagine tailoring cognitive training programs that are not only adapted to an individual's learning style but also to their genetic predisposition, maximizing the efficacy of the training based on genetic markers that predict neuroplastic responses.

Another exciting frontier is the integration of artificial intelligence with neuroplastic research. AI algorithms could be designed to predict the most effective learning and rehabilitation methods for any given individual, taking into account vast amounts of data on how different brain training exercises foster neuroplasticity. These AI systems could recommend daily activities that optimize cognitive function, adjust learning methods to prevent cognitive overload, and predict when a learner is ready to advance.

Finally, advancements in pharmacology promise to develop compounds that could enhance or accelerate neuroplastic responses. Specific drugs could be designed to increase the brain's plasticity temporarily, aiding in faster learning or recovery from injury. Such pharmacological supports would be used in conjunction with behavioral approaches to ensure the sustainability of cognitive gains.

With these advancements, the role of educators and therapists might transform significantly, shifting from conventional teaching and therapeutic methods to highly specialized and adaptive mediators of personalized brain development strategies. This not only would make learning more efficient and accessible but would also open new avenues for rehabilitating cognitive functions in patients with neurological conditions.

As we explore these potential advancements, it is clear that the intersection of technology, genetics, pharmacology, and cognitive science through the lens of neuroplasticity will not only deepen our understanding of the brain but could fundamentally enhance the human capacity to learn and adapt. The future of this research has the potential to transform educational systems and therapeutic practices, making cognitive enhancement a tailored, more effective component of daily life and health care.

Here are some MetaPrompts that revolve around the future advancements in neuroplasticity research and their applications in learning and cognitive enhancement:

[Advancements in Neuroimaging Techniques] - **Objective**: Explore the potential of advanced neuroimaging in enhancing personalized learning and therapy.
  - **ChatGPT MetaPrompt**: 'Generate a series of prompts to explore how future neuroimaging technologies could transform educational and therapeutic practices, including the development of real-time neural tracking systems.'
  - **Expected Output**: Prompts should guide users to consider scenarios, challenges, and benefits of implementing such technologies in real-world settings, focusing on case studies or hypothetical models.
  - **Follow Up**: Analyze responses to understand practical implications and ethical considerations, and refine the scenarios based on feedback to deepen the exploration.

[Genetic Influences on Neuroplasticity] - **Objective**: Investigate how genetic factors could be integrated into personalizing education and therapy.
  - **ChatGPT MetaPrompt**: 'Create prompts that ask about the ethical, practical, and scientific challenges of using genetic information to tailor cognitive training programs.'
  - **Expected Output**: Prompts should encourage discussions on privacy concerns, the accuracy of genetic testing, and the potential for personalized learning plans.
  - **Follow Up**: Gather various viewpoints to draft a comprehensive overview of public perception and scientific readiness for such a personalized approach.

[AI Integration in Neuroplastic Research] -

Objective: Discuss the role of artificial intelligence in predicting and enhancing cognitive functions.

   - **ChatGPT MetaPrompt**: 'Develop a set of prompts that invite users to brainstorm AI-driven solutions for optimizing neuroplastic training, highlighting both the opportunities and pitfalls.'

   - **Expected Output**: Prompts should lead to innovative ideas on AI configurations, potential biases in AI algorithms, and strategies to overcome these challenges.

   - **Follow Up**: Evaluate the feasibility of these ideas and assess how AI can be ethically and effectively implemented.

[**Pharmacological Advancements and Neuroplasticity**] - **Objective**: Examine how new drugs could support neuroplastic processes for faster learning and recovery.

   - **ChatGPT MetaPrompt**: 'Generate prompts that dive into the development, testing, and deployment of pharmacological agents designed to enhance neuroplastic responses.'

   - **Expected Output**: Discussion prompts focusing on clinical trials, FDA approval processes, and integration of pharmacology with existing therapies.

   - **Follow Up**: Use the insights from these discussions to create informative articles or presentations that can educate stakeholders about the potential impacts and challenges.

[**Transforming Roles of Educators and Therapists**] - **Objective**: Speculate on how future advances in neuroplasticity might redefine the professional responsibilities and methods of educators and therapists.

   - **ChatGPT MetaPrompt**: 'Create a sequence of prompts

that encourage detailed analysis of how the role of educators and therapists might evolve with the advances in neuroplasticity research.'

- **Expected Output**: The prompts should generate discussions on necessary training, potential shifts in educational curricula, and new therapeutic techniques.

- **Follow Up**: Compile the responses to inform policy recommendations and training programs for professionals adapting to these new roles.

These meta-prompts aim to foster a deeper understanding and critical examination of how the intersection of technology, genetics, pharmacology, and cognitive science through the lens of neuroplasticity can be harnessed to significantly enhance educational and therapeutic practices globally.

By executing these metaprompts, you will gain:

- **Enhanced Understanding of Neuroplasticity**: These prompts will deepen your comprehension of how advanced technologies and research are paving the way for significant innovations in the field of neuroplasticity. You'll grasp the complexities and potentials of integrating neuroimaging, genetics, AI, and pharmacology into learning and therapy.

- **Insight into Ethical and Practical Implications**: As you explore prompts focused on the ethical and practical aspects of these advancements, you will develop a nuanced perspective on the responsible use of genetic profiling, the implementation of AI in healthcare and education, and the ethical considerations in pharmacological enhancements.

- **Creative Problem-Solving Skills**: The metaprompts are designed to encourage brainstorming and problem-solving, helping you think critically about how to overcome challenges such as privacy concerns in genetic testing, biases in AI algorithms, or regulatory hurdles in drug approvals.

- **Opportunity for Innovation**: By prompting discussions on AI-driven solutions or genetic tailoring in cognitive training, you'll be at the forefront of conceptualizing innovative approaches that could revolutionize how we understand and enhance human cognitive functions.

- **Preparedness for Future Trends**: Engaging with these metaprompts will equip you with knowledge about the future direction of neuroplasticity research and its applications. This awareness is crucial for professionals in education, healthcare, and policy-making to stay ahead in their fields.

- **Collaborative Engagement**: These metaprompts encourage interaction and discussion, fostering a collaborative environment where ideas can be exchanged. This not only enhances personal knowledge but also contributes to a collective understanding that can drive societal and scientific progress.

- **Advocacy and Education**: Armed with in-depth knowledge and insights gained from addressing these prompts, you will be better prepared to advocate for ethical practices, informed policies, and public education about the benefits and limitations of emerging neuroplasticity technologies.

Executing these metaprompts isn't just about gaining information; it's about actively participating in the shaping of future educational and therapeutic frameworks that harness the power of neuroplasticity in ethically sound, scientifically validated, and highly personalized ways.

Neuroplasticity, with its profound capacity to reshape the neural pathways in response to various stimuli, holds remarkable implications for both educational strategies and cognitive health. As research continues to unravel how the brain adapts and reforms, our approach to learning and therapeutic interventions is poised for substantial transformation.

The insights gleaned from neuroplasticity research suggest a future where educational systems can customize learning experiences to the neural profiles of each student. This tailoring goes beyond traditional educational paradigms, potentially enabling a hyper-personalized learning environment that adjusts in real-time to optimize cognitive development based on an individual's response to various instructional strategies.

In terms of cognitive health, understanding neuroplasticity offers promising avenues for interventions in neurological disorders, aging, and cognitive decline. Therapeutic strategies could be designed to stimulate specific neural circuits, aiding recovery and enhancement of cognitive functions, thus significantly improving quality of life for individuals afflicted with cognitive impairments.

Reflecting on these prospects, it is evident that embracing neuroplasticity not only enriches our theoretical knowledge but also empowers us to devise more effective educational tools and therapeutic models. The ongoing exploration into the brain's plastic nature continues to break new ground, promising a future where learning is not just a process of acquiring information but an adaptive journey tailored to foster the unique potentials of every individual's brain. This adaptive approach does not merely adjust to cognitive needs; it anticipates and evolves with them, marking a new era in education and cognitive care.

NEUROPLASTICITY IN DISEASE AND RECOVERY

Neuroplasticity plays a fundamental role in both the development of various neurological conditions and the potential for recovery. This capacity of the brain to adapt — whether in the face of injury, disease, or environmental changes — brings profound implications for the field of neuroscience, shaping how we understand and approach recovery and rehabilitation. In diseases where the brain's adaptability might lead to undesirable outcomes, such as in chronic pain or certain mental health disorders, neuroplasticity can also signify hope, revealing pathways for therapeutic interventions that could reverse or mitigate these conditions.

This chapter dives into the dual-edged nature of neuroplasticity, examining how it can both contribute to and heal from neurological disorders. By dissecting how maladaptive neuroplastic changes might perpetuate conditions such as epilepsy, and how targeted therapeutic strategies can harness the brain's innate plasticity for recovery, this text aims to provide a comprehensive overview of the significant strides being made in this area. Each concept presented here is anchored in the latest research, illustrating the evolving strategies that leverage neuroplasticity for clinical benefit.

Understandably, the exploration of neuroplasticity is not just an academic endeavor; it is a topic of immense practical importance, offering innovative, impactful methods to support individuals suffering from neurological impairments. Through this chapter, readers will gain clear, actionable insights into how neuroplasticity influences both disease mechanics and recovery processes, framing a new narrative in neuroscience that fosters hope and promotes continual learning and adaptation.

Neuroplasticity, while often beneficial, can also play a pivotal role in the development of neurological disorders such as epilepsy and chronic pain. In epilepsy, neuroplasticity contributes to the formation of abnormal neural networks, where excessive and aberrant synaptic connectivity leads to recurrent seizures. This process can be likened to a computer system that has developed faulty connections, causing it to repeatedly crash under certain conditions. In the case of chronic pain, neuroplastic changes can lead to the nervous system becoming overly sensitive, amplifying pain signals without actual physical harm, much like a microphone that becomes too sensitive and picks up even the smallest noises as loud feedback.

Conversely, the same capacity of the brain to undergo plastic changes supports its ability to recover from these conditions. In epilepsy, treatments such as surgical interventions or therapeutic electrical stimulation aim to disrupt the maladaptive network connections and promote the formation of healthier patterns. This approach can be visualized as rewiring an electrical circuit to remove faulty connections and enhance the system's functionality.

For chronic pain, cognitive-behavioral therapies and

physical rehabilitation exploit neuroplasticity to 'retrain' the brain, dampening the heightened pain responses and promoting normal pain processing pathways. This process resembles tuning the microphone to normalize its sensitivity levels, thereby reducing the feedback it produces without necessary triggers.

Understanding the mechanisms of neuroplasticity in these disorders not only illuminates the root causes and perpetuation of such conditions but also opens avenues for innovative therapies that target the underlying plastic changes. Through this detailed exploration, one can appreciate the double-edged sword of neuroplasticity in neurological health—its role in both the development of debilitating conditions and the recovery processes that restore normal function.

Let's take a deeper look at the specific neural mechanisms of neuroplasticity involved in epilepsy and chronic pain, exploring how these mechanisms contribute to the conditions and how they can be targeted for recovery.

In epilepsy, abnormal synaptic connectivity is often at the heart of why seizures occur. This involves an imbalance between excitatory and inhibitory signals in the brain. Typically, excitatory neurotransmitters like glutamate and inhibitory neurotransmitters such as GABA (gamma-Aminobutyric acid) help maintain a balance in neural activity. However, in epilepsy, this balance is disrupted. Excessive activation of excitatory neurons or insufficient inhibition can lead to a hyperexcitable network where neurons fire too frequently and synchronously, leading to a seizure. This condition can be understood by examining the cells involved, primarily the pyramidal neurons in the cortex, known for their role in sending excitatory signals, and the various types of GABAergic interneurons that provide inhibitory feedback. The synaptic alterations might include changes in receptor density, altered ion channel function, or modifications in neurotransmitter uptake, each contributing to the erratic electrical activity characteristic of seizures.

Turning to chronic pain, treatments like cognitive-behavioral therapy (CBT) and physical rehabilitation work by modifying the pain pathways that neuroplasticity has maladaptively altered. Chronic pain often results from the nervous system's heightened sensitivity to pain signals, a condition often referred to as central sensitization. This involves an increase in the activity of neurons in the spinal cord that transmit pain signals to the brain. Through neuroplastic changes, non-painful stimuli can start triggering pain responses. CBT aims to 'rewire' these pain perceptions by altering the patient's emotional and cognitive response to pain, effectively reducing the brain's interpretation of these signals as painful. Physical rehabilitation, on the other hand, frequently engages in graded exercises which not only improve the physical condition but also encourage the brain to remap the correct responses to physical actions, gradually desensitizing the exaggerated pain responses.

Both treatments leverage the brain's inherent neuroplasticity—its ability to reform pathways and create new connections—to foster recovery. Understanding these molecular and cellular nuances provides profound insights into how adaptive and maladaptive neuroplastic mechanisms work within these health conditions. It underscores the potential therapies' ability to intercept and modify these pathways effectively, offering optimism for managing conditions traditionally deemed challenging. By incorporating this knowledge into therapeutic strategies, practitioners can significantly enhance the efficacy of treatment protocols, leading to better patient outcomes and an improved understanding of neural disorders in the broader medical context.

Imagine you're learning to dance, but instead of stepping onto a dance floor, you slip on a pair of virtual reality (VR) goggles and suddenly, you're in a ballroom. This scenario isn't far off from how virtual reality is being used in stroke rehabilitation. Just as a dance instructor guides your movements, VR systems guide stroke patients through therapies tailored to their physical capabilities, providing an immersive environment where they can practice movements and tasks.

In stroke rehabilitation, regaining motor skills can be as daunting as learning complex dance steps after years without practice. VR technology steps in as both a tutor and a practice partner. It creates a controlled, adaptable environment where patients can perform virtual tasks that mimic real-life activities—like picking up objects or walking down a street. This isn't just about going through the motions; it's about retraining the brain, leveraging the brain's plasticity which is its ability to reshape and learn new skills, even in adulthood.

The VR setup ensures that these exercises are not too easy

or too hard, much like a good dance instructor adjusts routines to match a student's progressing skill level. This customization ensures that patients are constantly challenged but not overwhelmed, optimizing the speed and effectiveness of their recovery. Real-time feedback, another cornerstone of VR therapy, acts like a mirror in a dance studio, allowing patients to adjust their movements and improve their technique.

Furthermore, the immersive nature of VR makes the rehabilitation process engaging, sometimes even enjoyable, combating the monotony that traditional therapies can entail. It's a blend of technology and healthcare, where patients get to 'play' their way to recovery, similar to how a child might learn to dance without realizing they're also enhancing their balance and coordination.

This approach to stroke rehabilitation highlights not only the innovation in therapeutic practices but also underscores the fundamental principle of neuroplasticity: the brain's remarkable ability to adapt and mend. It's a testament to the power of integrating technology with medical expertise to restore the quality of life and illustrates a future where recovery is not only about healing but also about re-engaging fully with the world.

Here is the breakdown of how virtual reality (VR) interfaces interact with the brain's neuroplastic capabilities in stroke rehabilitation:

- **<u>Types of VR Therapies</u>**:

- **Virtual Object Manipulation**: Engages patients in tasks like picking up, moving, and manipulating virtual objects, which mimics real-world hand and arm movements.
- **Navigational Tasks**: Involves moving through virtual environments, which helps improve spatial awareness and walking capabilities.
- **Balance Games**: Utilizes VR scenarios that challenge the patient's balance, aiding in the recovery of stability and posture.

- **Neurological Engagement**:
  - **Motor Cortex Stimulation**: VR tasks that require movement stimulate the motor cortex, enhancing the reconnection of neural pathways responsible for motor control.
  - **Sensory Feedback Activation**: Intensive sensory experiences in VR, such as visual or auditory elements of the virtual environment, activate corresponding sensory areas of the brain, promoting sensory integration and processing.
  - **Cognitive Function Engagement**: Problem-solving and strategy games in VR stimulate prefrontal cortex activities, improving cognitive functions that are often compromised in stroke patients.

- **Feedback Mechanisms**:
  - **Visual Feedback**: Provides real-time, visual cues that help patients correct posture, movement accuracy, and speed during rehabilitation exercises.
  - **Auditory Feedback**: Uses sounds to signal success or the need for adjustment, reinforcing the learning of correct movement patterns through auditory rewards.
  - **Haptic Feedback**: Delivers tactile responses through

VR controllers or suits, helping in the restoration of touch sensations and fine motor skills.

- **Customization and Adaptation**:
- **Progressive Difficulty Adjustment**: As the patient improves, VR systems increase the difficulty level of tasks automatically, ensuring that the patient continues to be challenged, fostering further neuroplasticity.
- **Task Variety**: VR systems can alter the types of tasks based on therapeutic needs and recovery progression, providing a wide range of activities to target different neural and motor functions.
- **Personalization**: VR rehabilitation programs are tailored to the individual's specific disabilities, personal goals, and progress, maximizing the efficacy of interventions based on neuroplastic principles of learning and adaptation.

This detailed exploration demonstrates how VR technologies harness and interact with neuroplasticity to support recovery in stroke rehabilitation. By continuously engaging various brain regions through immersive and interactive tasks, and adjusting to the user's progress, VR not only aids in the physical aspect of rehabilitation but also catalyzes the necessary neurobiological processes required for functional recovery and improvement.

Neurofeedback is a therapeutic intervention that leverages real-time displays of brain activity—often through EEG—to teach self-regulation of brain function to individuals with ADHD. It fundamentally operates on the principle of operant conditioning, a method where behaviors are modified based on their consequences. For instance, when patients successfully concentrate and reduce hyperactivity, they receive positive feedback such as points in a video game or changes in a music video, which are directly linked to their brainwave patterns. This process effectively trains them to enhance their attention and focus while reducing impulsivity by reinforcing neuroplastic changes in the brain's frontal cortex—the area associated with attention, decision-making, and impulse control.

Turning to brain-machine interfaces (BMIs), these devices have shown significant promise in restoring functions to individuals paralyzed due to spinal injuries or neurological disorders. BMIs typically read brain signals generated from the motor cortex and translate them into computer commands that operate external devices such as robotic arms or computer cursors. One of the most compelling uses has been to enable individuals with quadriplegia to control prosthetic limbs or regain control over their own limbs with the aid of powered exoskeletons. The technology harnesses the patient's intention to move, captured through neural activity, thereby enabling action.

Both technologies exemplify how understanding and manipulating brain activity can lead to substantial improvements in functions and quality of life. Neurofeedback and brain-machine interfaces not only demonstrate the adaptability and capabilities of the brain amidst dysfunction but also underscore the potential of these technologies to significantly alter therapeutic approaches and patient independence. However, the success and effectiveness of these interventions can vary greatly from one individual to another, highlighting a need for personalized approaches and further research to optimize their applications. This evolving field continues to push the boundaries of what medical science can achieve, offering hope and functional solutions where none existed before.

Neurofeedback systems and brain-machine interfaces (BMIs) are at the forefront of cutting-edge medical therapies, harnessing advanced technology to enhance patient outcomes. Let's explore the operational mechanisms that make these technologies essential tools in modern medicine.

Neurofeedback Systems:
1. **Configuration and Interpretation of EEG Data**:
 - Electroencephalography (EEG) systems are set up to capture electrical activity from the brain using sensors placed on the scalp. The raw signals are amplified and filtered to distinguish meaningful brainwave patterns from noise.
 - Interpretation of EEG data involves analyzing these wave patterns to identify specific frequencies and amplitudes associated with cognitive states. For instance, alpha waves might indicate relaxed wakefulness, while beta waves could denote active thinking or anxiety.

2. **Identifying and Linking EEG Patterns to Behavior**:
 - Machine learning algorithms are employed to correlate specific EEG patterns with behavioral outcomes. This is achieved by training the system on large datasets where known behaviors are matched with recorded EEG patterns.
 - For example, in treating ADHD, patterns indicating heightened focus might be linked to lower theta/beta wave ratios in the EEG data.

3. **Tailoring Feedback to Individual Needs**:
   - Once patterns are identified, personalized feedback mechanisms are programmed. This could be visual signals like a moving bar on the screen that the patient tries to control by maintaining concentration, or auditory feedback such as a tone that varies with brainwave activity.
   - Feedback is adjusted over sessions to fine-tune the responses, aiming to improve the patient's ability to self-regulate their brain functions over time.

Brain-Machine Interfaces (BMIs):
1. **Signal Acquisition through Neural Activity**:
   - BMIs start by using devices like microelectrode arrays implanted in the brain that record electrical signals from neurons. These signals are indicative of intentions or thought patterns related to movement or other functions.

2. **Signal Decoding Methodologies**:
   - Decoder algorithms are crucial. They interpret neural signals by distinguishing patterns that correspond to specific commands, like moving a cursor or a robotic limb.
   - Advanced signal processing techniques and machine learning paradigms are employed to enhance the accuracy and responsiveness of these decoders.

3. **System Calibration and Real-time Interaction**:
   - Calibration involves the user training with the system to refine the interfaces' ability to interpret their specific neural signatures correctly. This phase aligns the decoded signals with intended actions, ensuring the BMI outputs

match user intentions as closely as possible.

- In real-time operation, ongoing adjustments are made by the system to maintain synchronization between intended movements and the feedback from the prosthetic device or computer system, thus facilitating smoother control.

4. **<u>Role of Artificial Intelligence (AI)</u>**:
- AI plays a fundamental role in optimizing both neurofeedback and BMIs. In neurofeedback, AI algorithms adapt to changes in brain activity over time, improving the specificity of feedback. In BMIs, AI enhances decoding techniques, learning from each interaction to reduce the lag and error rates in interpreting neural signals.

- AI's adaptive learning capabilities ensure that these systems can evolve with the patient's progress, offering a truly personalized therapy experience.

By delving into these sophisticated operational mechanisms, one can appreciate how neurofeedback systems and BMIs utilize detailed neurocomputational strategies to transform medical therapy landscapes. This detailed exploration reveals the intricacies of how precisely controlled signals and feedback can lead to substantial improvements in treating conditions like ADHD and paralysis, illustrating the profound implications of integrating technology into therapeutic practices.

As we look toward the horizon of neuroplasticity research, exciting pioneering therapies like stem cell therapy and optogenetics hold the potential to dramatically transform the way neurological disorders are treated. Stem cell therapy, for instance, involves the introduction of new, healthy cells into damaged or diseased areas of the brain to repair or replace neural tissue. This approach could revolutionize treatments for conditions such as stroke or traumatic brain injuries, where lost or damaged neurons are the primary impediment to recovery. By fostering the growth of new neural pathways and enhancing the brain's ability to rewire itself, stem cell therapy offers a promising avenue to restore lost functions.

Optogenetics, on the other hand, uses light to control neurons that have been genetically modified to respond to specific wavelengths. This precision allows researchers to activate or inhibit distinct groups of neurons, offering insights into the neuronal activities underlying behaviors and pathological conditions. For therapeutic applications, optogenetics could be used to correct dysfunctional neural circuits, potentially providing relief for patients with neurological disorders such as Parkinson's disease or epilepsy.

Both of these innovative technologies leverage the principles of neuroplasticity—enhancing the brain's innate capability to adapt and morph. The precision of optogenetics and the regenerative potential of stem cell therapy could lead to highly targeted treatments that not only alleviate symptoms but also address the root causes of neurological diseases. As research advances, the integration of these technologies into clinical practice could usher in a new era of neurology, where brain repair and functional recovery are not just possibilities but realities. This not merely shifts the therapeutic paradigm but also offers hope to millions whose conditions were once deemed irreversible. As we continue to explore these frontier technologies, their full potential to reshape neurotherapeutic practices comes closer to being realized, marking a significant milestone in medical science and patient care.

Throughout this chapter, we have navigated the transformative landscape of neuroplasticity, unraveling how its principles are increasingly influencing medical and therapeutic advancements. From the integration of stem cell therapy in repairing brain damage to the precision of optogenetics in managing neurological disorders, the potential of neuroplasticity to mend and mold the human brain has been strikingly evident.

We dived into how these innovative therapies not only promise to alleviate symptoms but also aim to address the root causes of neurological conditions by harnessing the brain's innate ability to reorganize itself. The exploration underlined the emergence of treatments that go beyond mere symptom management, offering prospects for substantial recovery and enhancement of life quality for individuals afflicted with neurological conditions.

As we look to the future, the importance of adopting and integrating neuroplastic principles into new medical enhancements cannot be overstated. The ongoing research and clinical trials in neuroplasticity not only pave the way for revolutionary treatments but also promise to redefine the boundaries of what is medically achievable. This calls for a sustained commitment to research and innovation in this field, ensuring that the insights gained from neuroplasticity can be fully harnessed to remodel therapeutic practices and patient care.

In conclusion, as we continue to advance our understanding and application of neuroplastic principles, the horizon of neurology and rehabilitation is set to expand dramatically. These advancements hold the key to unlocking treatments that could fundamentally alter the course of recovery for numerous neurological afflictions, marking a new era of hope and possibility in healthcare.

AGE AND NEUROPLASTICITY

The brain's remarkable ability to form and reorganize synaptic connections in response to learning or experience, holds a pivotal role as we age. This chapter, 'Age and Neuroplasticity,' addresses how changes in neuroplasticity can affect cognitive functions as we grow older and explores interventions that can help mitigate the effects of aging on the brain. An understanding of neuroplasticity not only illuminates why certain cognitive functions might decline with age but also reveals how lifelong learning and certain therapies can maintain—even improve—cognitive agility despite advancing years.

By examining how neuroplastic responses change over a lifetime, this chapter underscores the substantial influence that nurturing our neuronal pathways can have on extending cognitive vitality. Insight into this aspect of brain health provides not only hope but also practical strategies for aging individuals to sustain their mental acuity. Thus, cultivating a robust understanding of neuroplasticity empowers us to actively shape our brain's aging process, transforming the way we approach mental decline and cognitive rehabilitation in older adults. Here, you will find a concise exploration into the dynamic interactions between aging and neuroplasticity, offering valuable knowledge on maintaining cognitive health through various stages of life.

Engage with this chapter to navigate the complexities of

aging intertwined with neuroplastic possibilities, unraveling how targeted neuroplastic interventions can substantially enrich the lives of the elderly.

Neuroplasticity refers to the brain's ability to reorganize itself by forming new neural connections throughout a person's life. This ability allows the brain to adjust its activities in response to new situations or changes in one's environment. Think of the brain as a dynamic map filled with roads and pathways; neuroplasticity represents the construction, modification, and removal of these roads and paths to enable efficient communication across various areas of the brain.

In youth, the brain exhibits a high degree of plasticity, making it extremely responsive to learning and experience. During these early years, much like a city in rapid development, the brain's neural pathways are highly dynamic, forming and reconfiguring at an impressive rate. This fluidity allows for the swift acquisition of new skills and abilities. As one ages, these pathways become more established—similar to well-trodden paths in a mature city. While the brain retains the ability to adapt and change, these changes occur at a slower pace and require more effort.

For individuals, understanding neuroplasticity emphasizes the importance of continuously engaging in mentally stimulating activities that challenge the brain, which can help maintain cognitive agility and memory as they age. For medical practitioners, it underscores the need for therapies that support or enhance neuroplasticity, especially in treating conditions like stroke or dementia, where enhancing the brain's ability to form new connections can be critical for recovery and rehabilitation.

This insight into how neuroplasticity functions is crucial, not just for academic or medical interests but for practical application in daily life and health. It promotes a proactive approach to both personal mental health and broader medical practices. This knowledge equips both individuals and health professionals with the tools to foster a healthier, more adaptable brain regardless of age.

Let's take a deeper look at the fascinating world of neuroplasticity by exploring the cellular and molecular mechanisms that enable this incredible brain adaptability. Neuroplasticity is primarily concerned with the changes that occur at neuron connections, known as synapses, which allow for the transmission and modulation of electrical and chemical signals between neurons.

Firstly, synaptic plasticity is a core component of neuroplasticity. It includes mechanisms like long-term potentiation (LTP) and long-term depression (LTD), which are vital for learning and memory. LTP enhances the strength of synaptic connections following repeated stimulation, essentially making it easier for neurons to transmit signals to each other. This process involves the increase of neurotransmitter release or the density of neurotransmitter receptors at the synapse. In contrast, LTD reduces synaptic strength, acting as a necessary balance and refinement mechanism, preventing the over-excitation of neuronal circuits, which can be detrimental.

Neurotransmitters—chemicals such as glutamate, dopamine, and serotonin—play pivotal roles in these processes. Glutamate, for instance, is crucial for LTP. It activates NMDA receptors at synapses, leading to a cascade of signals that ultimately result in the strengthening of the synaptic connection. Dopamine and serotonin can modulate these pathways, influencing both the mood and the efficacy of learning mechanisms.

As we age, these processes can become less efficient. The brain loses some of its synaptic connections, and the remaining synapses may not adjust as easily to new information or stimuli. This decline is partly why learning new skills or remembering information can become more challenging as we grow older.

To counter these effects, specific therapeutic techniques have been developed to enhance neuroplasticity. Cognitive training exercises, for instance, are designed to consistently challenge the brain, thereby fostering new synaptic connections. These exercises might involve tasks that require problem-solving, memory recall, or learning new information—all aimed at stimulating synaptic plasticity.

Similarly, physical therapy plays a crucial role, especially in individuals recovering from neural injuries. Movements and physical exercises can trigger the release of various neurotrophic factors, chemicals that support neuron growth and the strengthening of synapses, thereby enhancing the brain's ability to rewire itself.

The biochemical and physiological impacts of these therapies are profound. They not only help in maintaining synaptic flexibility but also in mitigating the natural decline of neuroplasticity with age. By continually engaging in these therapies, older adults can better maintain their cognitive agility and delay the onset of age-related cognitive impairments.

Understanding these intricate cellular and molecular mechanisms not only provides insight into the brain's adaptability but also underscores the importance of active engagement in cognitively and physically stimulating activities. It's a testimony to the principle that at any age, the brain is capable of remarkable adjustments, fundamentally shaping our interaction with the world around us.

Imagine the brain's ability to adapt and reorganize itself—known as neuroplasticity—as a garden at different stages of growth. In young brains, neuroplasticity is like a budding plant, sprouting with vibrant, flexible stems that easily bend and stretch towards the sunlight. This flexibility represents the youthful brain's ability to rapidly form new connections, allowing it to quickly learn new skills and recover from injuries. The process is natural and almost effortless, much like how young shoots grow and adapt to their environment.

Contrast this with an older brain, which can be likened to an established, mature tree. The tree's sturdy, thick branches are not as pliable as the young plant's stems. They grow more slowly and are less likely to adapt their shape to immediate surroundings. Similarly, as we age, our brain's neuroplastic capabilities, though still present, become more rigid. Making new neural connections in an older brain requires more time and a greater number of repeated actions and learning efforts. This doesn't mean the tree—or the aging brain—can't grow or adjust at all, but the process is not as swift or as fluid as in its younger counterpart.

The differences in neuroplasticity between the younger and older brains affect how each responds to new challenges or injuries. While the younger brain can quickly reroute around damaged areas, using its high plasticity to minimize disruptions caused by injury, the older brain may struggle to find new pathways, making recovery a longer and more complex process.

Understanding this shift in neuroplastic capabilities from the sprightly flexibility of youth to the more deliberate growth of age highlights the critical need to engage continually in activities that promote mental flexibility. For younger individuals, it validates the enrichment of their cognitive landscapes through varied learning experiences. For older adults, it underscores the importance of maintaining cognitive exercises to nurture and sustain their mental agility. Just as a gardener carefully tends to both the young plant and the old tree, tending to our brain's health throughout life can keep it as enriched and responsive as possible. Thus, appreciating and nurturing our neuroplasticity is essential for our brain's lifelong health and adaptability.

Here is the breakdown of the biological and molecular mechanisms underlying neuroplasticity, providing an enhanced understanding of how the brain adapts throughout different life stages:

- **Neural Pathway Formation**:
  - **Early Development**: During early development, neurons in the brain rapidly form new connections. This prolific phase, largely driven by genetic instructions and early sensory experiences, sets up the basic architecture of the brain.
  - **Synaptogenesis**: This is the process where neurons form synapses with each other, enabling them to communicate through electrochemical signals.
  - **Pruning**: As the infant grows, less used synapses are pruned away, which makes the neural network more efficient, based on the "use it or lose it" principle.
  - **Changes with Age**: As we age, the rate of forming new neuronal connections slows down, but the potential for forming new connections, or neurogenesis, continues, although at a reduced pace.
  - **Regulatory changes**: The brain continues to create neurons and synapses but does this more in response to learning and memory tasks or recovery from injury.

- **Synaptic Strength Changes**:
  - **Strengthening (Long-Term Potentiation, LTP)**: LTP involves the strengthening of synapses based on increased activity and is crucial for learning and memory.
  - **Role of Glutamate**: Glutamate receptors, especially NMDA receptors, play a key role in LTP. Activation of these receptors leads to calcium influx and subsequent signaling pathways that enhance synaptic strength.
  - **Weakening (Long-Term Depression, LTD)**:

Conversely, LTD involves the weakening of synaptic connections through decreased synaptic activity.

- **Role of GABA**: GABAergic signaling contributes to LTD by inhibiting neuronal activity thereby scaling down unnecessary or weak synaptic connections.

- **Molecular Factors**:
  - **Brain-Derived Neurotrophic Factor (BDNF)**: BDNF is crucial in supporting the survival of existing neurons and the growth of new neurons and synapses.
    - **Changes with Age**: Levels of BDNF can decrease with age, leading to diminished neuroplasticity. However, activities like exercise and cognitive challenges can help maintain or elevate BDNF levels.

- **Impact of Environmental Stimuli**:
  - **Enhancement by Positive Stimuli**: Learning new skills, physical exercise, and rich social interactions can enhance brain plasticity by fostering new synaptic connections and releasing growth factors.
    - **Cognitive Resilience**: Continuous engagement in intellectually challenging activities builds cognitive reserve, helping to maintain brain function as aging progresses.
  - **Impairment by Negative Stimuli**: Chronic stress, isolation, and poor diet can impair neuroplasticity.
    - **Stress and Cortisol**: Prolonged exposure to cortisol, a stress hormone, can damage the hippocampus and impair the formation of new neurons, affecting memory and learning abilities.

This comprehensive look into the mechanisms of neuroplasticity reveals the intricate ballet of biological processes that allow the brain to adapt from infancy through old age. By understanding and influencing these processes, we can better support brain health across all stages of life.

Reduced neuroplasticity in aging individuals presents notable challenges, primarily manifesting as slower learning rates and extended recovery periods from cognitive impairments. As neuroplasticity declines, the brain's ability to form new neural connections diminishes, which is crucial for learning new skills and information. This change can liken to a well-worn path becoming overgrown; the familiar route remains, but creating new paths becomes increasingly laborious.

This decline impacts everyday learning scenarios. For instance, an older adult learning to use a new technology might need more repetitions to familiarize themselves with the process compared to a younger person. Similarly, recovery from neurological events like strokes can be prolonged because the brain's capacity to rewire itself and compensate for damaged areas is not as robust.

To address these challenges, several modern strategies have been developed to enhance cognitive flexibility in older adults. One effective approach is cognitive training, which involves tasks designed to improve specific cognitive functions. These exercises can range from simple memory games to complex problem-solving tasks, all aimed at stimulating neuroplasticity.

Physical activity also plays a crucial role. Regular exercise, particularly aerobic workouts, has been shown to increase the production of brain-derived neurotrophic factor (BDNF), a protein that supports the growth and differentiation of new neurons and synapses. BDNF essentially acts as a fertilizer for the brain, promoting growth and resilience at the cellular level.

Additionally, social engagement and a healthy diet rich in antioxidants are vital. Social interactions stimulate the brain through diverse and complex conversations, while antioxidants reduce oxidative stress, a factor that can impede neuronal function.

Together, these strategies form a comprehensive approach to tackling the limitations posed by reduced neuroplasticity in the aging population. By integrating these tactics into daily routines, older adults can better maintain cognitive agility, mitigating the impacts of age-related declines in brain function. Each of these strategies not only supports the brain's intrinsic abilities to adapt and reorganize but also highlights a proactive stance on aging, portraying it as a phase of life where growth and adaptation are still very much achievable.

Step-by-Step Guide: Enhancing Neuroplasticity in Older Adults

1. Cognitive Training:
- **Stimulating Synaptic Growth and Neuronal Activity**: Regular mental challenges such as puzzles, learning a new language, or playing musical instruments work to

increase neural activity. This activity encourages the growth of new synaptic connections and strengthens existing ones, a process critical for neuroplasticity.

- **Impact on Cognitive Functions**: These activities primarily benefit functions like memory, problem-solving, and multitasking abilities. Engaging in these exercises helps maintain and even improve these cognitive functions by regularly 'exercising' the relevant neural circuits, much like muscle strength improves with physical exercise.

2. Physical Exercise:
- **Increasing BDNF Levels**: Aerobic exercises, such as walking, swimming, or cycling, enhance the production of Brain-Derived Neurotrophic Factor (BDNF). BDNF is a critical protein that supports the survival of existing neurons and encourages the growth of new neurons and synapses.
- **Biochemical Support for Neurogenesis and Synaptic Plasticity**: The increase in BDNF not only promotes the formation of new neural pathways but also helps in the repair and protection of existing brain cells. This biochemical enhancement is vital for sustaining the brain's capacity to adapt, which is particularly important as natural regenerative processes slow with age.

3. Social Engagement:
- **Diverse Neuronal Stimulation**: Social interactions require the brain to process complex auditory and emotional cues, stimulating diverse areas of the brain. Regular, meaningful conversations can enhance cognitive flexibility and depth by engaging multiple neural pathways.
- **Neural Pathways Involved**: The primary areas involved include the temporal and frontal lobes which

handle language processing and emotional regulation. By actively participating in social settings, older adults can keep these critical regions of the brain engaged and functional, helping to preserve and enhance these functions.

Connecting Activities to Improved Brain Function:

Each of these activities contributes to maintaining the structural integrity and functional capacity of the brain. By understanding how cognitive training, physical exercise, and social engagement each biologically affect the brain, older adults and caregivers can better appreciate their significance. More importantly, this understanding provides a strong motivation to integrate these activities into daily routines, aiming to achieve a more resilient and adaptive brain despite the challenges of aging.

This guide emphasizes that maintaining an active lifestyle, both mentally and physically, can have profound benefits for the brain's health and capabilities, ultimately leading to a higher quality of life in older age.

Imagine trying to run the latest software on an old computer: it might struggle, dragging its virtual feet, much like the aging brain can falter under the demands of retaining new information and maintaining cognitive agility. Current and emerging therapies aimed at boosting neuroplasticity in older adults are similar to not just upgrading the operating system of an old computer, but also installing more RAM and a new, faster processor to revitalize its efficiency and responsiveness.

One such 'hardware upgrade' for the brain comes in the form of cognitive training programs, designed specifically to enhance mental flexibility and memory. Think of these as sophisticated, tailor-made software designed to defragment the brain and organize data more efficiently, allowing for quicker access and better usability.

Physical exercise can be viewed as adding a new cooling system to prevent the machine from overheating, or perhaps increasing its power supply. Regular physical activity promotes the release of proteins like BDNF (brain-derived neurotrophic factor), acting like a performance-enhancing tuning kit that helps the brain generate new cells and connections.

Additionally, modern pharmacological interventions, which aim at fine-tuning the neurological pathways, much like optimizing a computer's background processes, can help manage and mitigate the decline in brain plasticity. These drugs adjust the complex chemical neurotransmitters, streamlining the communication between neurons to maintain and enhance cognitive functions.

Social engagement, meanwhile, equips the old system with the latest in network cards, enabling better connections to external devices—in this case, other human brains. This social connection stimulates the brain, much like how high-speed internet allows for rapid information processing and acquisition, improving overall cognitive processing.

Through these therapies—be it neural 'hardware'

enhancements or 'software' updates—geriatric neuroplasticity is given a new lease on life, demonstrating that an older brain, much like an old computer, can indeed learn new tricks and run more efficiently with the right kind of modifications. These strategies not only extend the functional lifespan of the brain but also ensure that later years can be enjoyed with a sharper, more responsive mind.

Here's what we accomplish by executing all the prompts:

- **Understanding Neuroplasticity**: Grasp the basic and advanced concepts of how neuroplasticity works.

- **Cognitive Training Insight**: Learn specific cognitive exercises and how they directly enhance mental faculties such as memory and problem-solving.

- **Physical Health Connections**: Discover how physical exercises influence brain chemistry to support neuroplasticity, particularly through the release of BDNF.

- **Dietary Impacts**: Explore how certain nutrients and dietary patterns affect brain health and contribute to maintaining and enhancing cognitive functions.

- **Mental Health**: Understand the relationship between mental health and brain plasticity, emphasizing preventative and active care strategies.

- **Technological and Pharmacological Advances**: Get acquainted with how current technology and medications can be harnessed to enhance brain function and counteract the effects of aging on the brain.

- **Social Engagement**: Learn about the cognitive benefits of maintaining active social connections and how they stimulate neuroplasticity.

Each prompt not only serves as a learning tool but also enables you to implement practical steps towards maintaining or improving neuroplasticity in the context of aging. This set of customized prompts will guide you through understanding and eventually mastering the art of employing various strategies to keep the aging brain active and healthy.

Emerging research areas and technological innovations hold promising potentials for deepening our understanding and enhancing neuroplasticity in aging brains, particularly with the integration of artificial intelligence (AI) and machine learning. One of the promising aspects, for instance, involves the use of AI to analyze vast amounts of neurological data rapidly and accurately. AI algorithms can detect patterns and changes in brain activity that might elude human researchers, helping to identify signs of declining neuroplasticity much earlier. This capability enables a more proactive approach to managing aging-related cognitive decline.

Further, machine learning models can be trained to personalize cognitive training programs. By analyzing the initial capabilities and progress of an individual, these models can adjust the difficulty and type of cognitive exercises provided, optimizing the effectiveness of the training for enhancing neuroplasticity. This personalized approach can significantly improve outcomes, making cognitive enhancement efforts more effective and tailored to individual needs.

Additionally, the advent of brain-computer interfaces (BCIs) enhanced by machine learning algorithms offers another innovative frontier. BCIs could potentially enable direct stimulation of specific brain areas to enhance neuroplasticity. With machine learning, these interfaces could evolve to become more intuitive and efficient, eventually learning to adapt real-time to the user's neurological responses, thus providing custom stimuli that foster maximum neuroplastic enhancement.

However, while these technological advancements promise significant strides in the field, they come with their complexities. For example, the ethics of AI and data privacy, particularly concerning personal medical data, remain a crucial consideration. Moreover, the integration of these technologies into mainstream medical practice requires substantial validation to ensure safety and efficacy.

To stay abreast of these advancements, one might consider regularly reviewing published research and participating in forums dedicated to neuroplasticity and technological innovations in neuroscience. Engaging with these resources will not only improve understanding but also ensure that one is well-informed about the latest developments and their practical applications to enhancing neuroplasticity in aging brains. This approach ensures a strategic advantage in harnessing technology to manage and potentially reverse age-related cognitive declines effectively.

The exploration of age and neuroplasticity reveals a dynamic and evolving landscape where ongoing research and innovative therapeutic approaches promise enhanced life quality in older age. As we understand more about how the brain's ability to adapt and change declines with age, scientists and clinicians are developing methods to bolster neuroplasticity through targeted therapies and lifestyle interventions. These advances, which include everything from cognitive training programs tailored to individual needs to pharmacological treatments that enhance synaptic plasticity, are making it increasingly possible to counteract the age-related deterioration of mental faculties.

Moreover, the integration of cutting-edge technologies such as machine learning and brain-computer interfaces into these therapeutic strategies provides a highly personalized approach to cognitive enhancement. Such tools not only offer refined methods to stimulate brain activity but also equip medical practitioners with more accurate and effective means to diagnose, assess, and treat neuroplastic declines in older adults. This emphasis on customization in therapy acknowledges and addresses the variation in neuroplasticity among individuals, ensuring that the interventions are as effective as possible.

These developments in neuroplasticity research signify a profound shift in how we approach aging and cognitive health. Far from accepting cognitive decline as an inevitable part of aging, the scientific community is fostering optimism that aging individuals can maintain, and even improve, their mental agility. By continuing to support and pay attention to this research, society can better prepare to meet the needs of its aging population, ensuring that more people enjoy not just longer but more cognitively vibrant lives. These efforts not only enhance the lives of older adults but also enrich the communities they are part of, creating a deeply positive impact on society as a whole.

TECHNOLOGICAL AND THERAPEUTIC ADVANCES

In the dynamic field of neuroscience, technological and therapeutic advances are profoundly reshaping our understanding of neuroplasticity—the brain's remarkable ability to reorganize itself by forming new neural connections throughout an individual's life. These innovations are not merely academic; they offer real-world applications that promise substantial improvements in treating brain disorders and enhancing cognitive functions. This chapter lays a clear foundation, explaining how cutting-edge tools and methods like transcranial magnetic stimulation and cognitive behavioral therapies leverage neuroplasticity to provide tailored treatment solutions. Each section will build upon this premise, presenting the information in a straightforward manner that demystifies complex scientific concepts and makes them accessible and relevant. Our exploration will bridge the gap between intricate neurological processes and their practical applications in medicine, providing you with a thorough understanding of how modern science is transforming the landscape of brain health and therapy. This breakdown not only informs but also illuminates the significant impact these advances hold for the future of medical science and patient care.

Neuroplasticity refers to the brain's incredible ability to adapt and rewire itself by forming new neural connections. This capacity is crucial not only during early developmental stages but throughout an individual's life, responding to learning, experience, and injury. Fundamentally, it involves the strengthening or weakening of existing connections or even the creation of entirely new pathways that affect how information flows in the brain.

In the context of medical treatment, this adaptability holds transformative potential. For instance, neuroplasticity is at the heart of recovery strategies for stroke survivors, where therapies focus on retraining the brain to regain functions, such as speech and mobility, which might have been compromised. Therapeutic exercises are designed to engage and strengthen other parts of the brain to take over the functions of the damaged areas, essentially reprogramming the brain's circuitry.

Moreover, the principles of neuroplasticity are driving the development of innovative neurological therapies. Technologies like transcranial magnetic stimulation, which non-invasively stimulates specific brain regions, leverage neuroplasticity to alter neuronal activity and have shown promise in treating conditions ranging from depression to Parkinson's disease. These interventions, by effectively 'rewiring' the brain, help mitigate symptoms and improve cognitive functions in conditions that were once considered immutable.

Understanding neuroplasticity thus not only deepens our comprehension of brain functionality but also expands the horizons for treating a spectrum of neurological disorders. By continuing to explore how the brain can be guided to reshape itself, researchers and clinicians are uncovering new, more effective ways to enhance brain health and rectify neurological impairments. This exploration also challenges and refines our conceptions of recovery and health, emphasizing an adaptable and fundamentally optimistic view of the human brain.

Neuroplasticity is the brain's ability to reorganize itself by forming new neural connections throughout life. This guide offers a detailed understanding of the biological mechanisms that underpin this fundamental aspect of brain function and how it is harnessed in various therapeutic settings.

1. **Synaptic Plasticity**

Synaptic plasticity refers to the ability of synapses, the points where nerve cells connect, to strengthen or weaken over time in response to increases or decreases in their activity. When a neuron is consistently stimulated, the synaptic connection it forms with another neuron becomes stronger. This is often referred to as "Long-Term Potentiation" or LTP, a process that involves various neurotransmitters, notably glutamate, and an increase in calcium ion concentration in the receiving neuron. Conversely, when synaptic activity is reduced, the connection weakens, known as "Long-Term Depression" (LTD). This dynamic adjusting of synaptic strength is critical for learning and memory. Additionally, synaptic pruning, the process of removing weaker synaptic contacts, plays a crucial role in refining neural connections and enhancing the efficiency of neuronal transmissions.

2. **Neural Adaptability**

Following an injury, the brain engages in a reorganization process, making new connections and sometimes even using alternative neural pathways to compensate for lost functions. Neurotrophic factors, particularly Brain-Derived Neurotrophic Factor (BDNF), play a vital role in this adaptability. BDNF supports the survival of existing neurons and encourages the growth and differentiation of new neurons and synapses. This factor is crucial in brain recovery processes following traumatic or ischemic injuries like stroke.

3. **Application in Therapies**

Transcranial Magnetic Stimulation (TMS) is a non-invasive technique used to modulate neural activities in targeted brain regions. This technology utilizes magnetic fields to induce small electric currents, stimulating neurons in the brain. The action of TMS can enhance or suppress brain activities, depending on the frequency of the magnetic pulses used. Such modulation can lead to improved cognitive functions or alleviation of psychiatric symptoms, underlining its therapeutic potential in conditions such as depression or Parkinson's disease.

4. **Examples of Neuroplasticity in Action**

A practical illustration of neuroplasticity involves the rehabilitation of stroke survivors. Through physical therapy and cognitive training exercises, patients relearn basic functions such as walking or speech. These therapies often involve repetitive tasks that encourage the brain to rewire and make new connections, compensating for the areas that have been damaged. This process is facilitated by the brain's plastic nature, driven by activities specifically designed to target and improve specific neurological deficits.

This comprehensive look into neuroplasticity not only illuminates the scientific backdrop of brain adaptability but links these concepts with real-world applications, underscoring the profound impact of ongoing research in shaping effective therapies. Through this understanding, one can fully appreciate the capacity of the human brain to adapt and overcome, providing a basis for the development of further innovations in neurological therapies.

Imagine you have a complex network of electrical wiring in your house that sometimes needs a tune-up to work more efficiently or to fix specific issues—it's somewhat similar with our brain circuits. Transcranial Magnetic Stimulation (TMS) and Deep Brain Stimulation (DBS) are like sophisticated electricians specially trained to fine-tune our brain's electrical activities.

TMS works from the outside, much like adjusting a home's electrical panel without invasive wiring changes. A magnetic coil placed near the head generates brief magnetic pulses, which pass effortlessly through the skull to stimulate or modulate brain activity underneath. This can be likened to using a remote control to adjust the volume on your stereo, enhancing or reducing the intensity as needed. It's particularly helpful for conditions like depression, where certain brain areas need a 'boost' to their electrical activity.

On the other hand, DBS is similar to installing a smart

thermostat directly into your home's heating system for more precise control. During DBS, surgeons implant tiny electrodes in specific areas of the brain. These electrodes are connected to a battery-operated device placed in the chest, which sends electrical impulses to the brain. Think of it as fine-tuning your home's temperature by making small adjustments directly at the source, which can be crucial for managing conditions like Parkinson's disease where specific areas of the brain circuitry require direct and ongoing adjustments.

Both of these techniques, therefore, offer powerful ways to 'rewire' the brain's electrical connections for better functionality. They highlight not just our growing understanding of brain functionality but also our increasing ability to influence it positively. By applying these sophisticated methods, medical professionals can help improve the quality of life for individuals with various neurological conditions, demonstrating a meaningful application of how adjusting the brain's electrical wiring can enhance its overall performance.

Here is the detailed breakdown on the mechanisms of action for Transcranial Magnetic Stimulation (TMS) and Deep Brain Stimulation (DBS), focusing on their impacts at the cellular and molecular levels and their therapeutic utility in treating neurological disorders:

- **Transcranial Magnetic Stimulation (TMS)**:
  - **Mechanism of Action**:
    - **Magnetic Coil Function**: A magnetic coil placed near the scalp generates brief magnetic pulses. These pulses

induce small electric fields in the underlying brain tissue.
- **Interaction with Neuronal Membranes**: The electric fields generated by these pulses interact with the neuronal membranes, temporarily altering the electrical environment of the neurons.
  - **Impact on Neurons**:
  - **Depolarization of Neurons**: The induced electric field can cause depolarization of neurons, leading to the generation of an action potential if the depolarization threshold is reached.
  - **Neurotransmitter Release**: Following depolarization, neurons release neurotransmitters into the synaptic cleft, which can enhance or inhibit the activity of post-synaptic neurons.
  - **Synaptic Plasticity**: Repeated stimulation can lead to long-term potentiation or depression of synaptic strength, which is critical for adaptive changes in brain activity.
  - **Therapeutic Applications**:
  - **Treatment of Depression**: By targeting regions like the prefrontal cortex, TMS can modulate the activity in neural circuits that are dysfunctional in depression, thereby alleviating symptoms.
  - **Other Conditions**: TMS is also being explored for its effectiveness in treating conditions like anxiety disorders, PTSD, and schizophrenia.

- **Deep Brain Stimulation (DBS)**:
  - **Surgical Installation**:
  - **Electrode Placement**: Electrodes are surgically implanted into specific brain regions, typically targeting areas that control movement, such as the subthalamic nucleus or globus pallidus.
  - **Target Regions**: The regions are selected based on

the disorder being treated and the desired modulation effect on brain circuits.
   - **Neuronal Stimulation**:
   - **Electrical Impulses**: A battery-operated device, commonly placed under the skin of the chest, sends electrical impulses through the electrodes directly into brain tissues.
   - **Influence on Neurons**: These impulses can modulate neuronal activity, either by exciting or inhibiting neurons, based on the frequency of stimulation.
   - **Therapeutic Applications**:
   - **Parkinson's Disease**: DBS helps in managing symptoms such as tremors, stiffness, and difficulty with movement by modulating the motor circuits.
   - **Extension to Other Disorders**: Beyond movement disorders, DBS is also being researched for its potential benefits in epilepsy, obsessive-compulsive disorder, and major depressive disorder.

This comprehensive overview not only discusses how TMS and DBS operate on a technical level but also clarifies why these treatments are effectively used for specific neurological conditions, enhancing our understanding of their clinical relevance.

The application of Artificial Intelligence (AI) in customizing cognitive therapy is a pivotal advancement in enhancing neuroplasticity, tailored specifically to the needs and performance of individual patients. AI systems analyze large datasets of patient interactions and responses during cognitive training sessions, identifying patterns and learning rates unique to each individual. This data-driven approach allows therapists to adjust the difficulty and types of tasks in real time, effectively targeting the neural circuits most in need of intervention.

For instance, if a patient is undergoing cognitive rehabilitation after a stroke, AI can monitor their progress across various tasks like memory games or problem-solving activities. It assesses not just accuracies but the time taken and the cognitive load, adjusting the upcoming tasks to either escalate challenges or reinforce current skills based on real-time data. This customization ensures that every session is optimized for maximum therapeutic effect, encouraging neural adaptation and growth.

Moreover, AI's ability to continually learn and adapt its algorithms based on new data means that the therapy remains as effective as possible even as the patient's capabilities evolve. This is crucial for sustaining engagement and progress, particularly in neuroplasticity where repeated, targeted brain activity is necessary for recovery and improvement.

One of the challenges, however, lies in ensuring that the AI systems are accessible and interpretable by healthcare providers who may not have specialized knowledge in AI technology. Therefore, the design of these AI systems often includes user-friendly interfaces that present data analyses and suggestions in an understandable format, enabling therapists to make informed decisions about patient care.

This sophisticated use of AI not only deepens our understanding of individual differences in cognitive therapy but also significantly enhances the ability to provide personalized care that adapates to an individual's therapeutic needs. Thus, AI in cognitive therapy not only represents a technical achievement but also a substantial leap forward in making neuroplasticity-based treatments more effective and responsive.

Let's take a detailed look at how Artificial Intelligence (AI) operates in analyzing patient data during cognitive therapy sessions to enhance neuroplasticity, ensuring each concept is as clear as if it were being explained over coffee:

- **Data Collection**:
AI systems in cognitive therapy gather various types of data that include reaction times which show how quickly a person responds to a task, accuracy rates which reflect the correctness of the responses, and different types of errors which help in understanding the areas where the patient struggles. These data points are crucial as they provide a comprehensive view of a patient's cognitive performance and progression over time.

- **Pattern Recognition**:
To identify patterns and learning rates from this collected data, sophisticated algorithms such as neural networks and machine learning classifiers are employed. Neural networks, which mimic the structure of human brain cells, are adept at recognizing complex patterns from vast datasets. These networks adjust their internal parameters based on the correction of errors in prediction, improving

their accuracy over time. Meanwhile, machine learning classifiers categorize data based on input features, such as distinguishing between successful and unsuccessful task completions, to predict outcomes and learning rates.

- **Real-Time Adjustments**:

From the insights gained through pattern recognition, AI decides on real-time adjustments to the therapeutic regime. If a patient shows improvement, the AI can escalate the difficulty of tasks to challenge the patient further. Conversely, if a patient is struggling, it might reinforce current skills by repeating similar tasks or reducing complexity. This decision-making process is driven by predefined thresholds of performance metrics and predictive analytics which forecast likely outcomes based on current trends in the data.

- **Interface Design**:

The clarity and usability of the AI system's user interface for therapists are paramount. It involves employing user-friendly design principles that allow straightforward navigation and manipulation of the therapy parameters. Good interface design will also include effective data visualization techniques, showing patient progress with clear graphs, and color-coded alert systems to draw attention to important changes or areas needing focus. Interaction design principles ensure that the system is responsive and adaptable to therapist input, making the tool as intuitive as possible, thereby reducing the cognitive load on the therapist.

By dissecting the AI-driven processes in cognitive therapy

into these components, it becomes evident how technology not only supports but actively enhances the effectiveness of treatments catered to individual neuroplasticity needs. This deeper understanding stamps the importance of AI in the dynamic field of cognitive therapeutic interventions, making it an invaluable asset in the pursuit of personalized medicine.

Neuroplasticity-based technologies and therapies have revolutionized treatment approaches for various neurological disorders, providing hope and substantial improvements in many patients' lives. Here, we explore a few case studies that highlight the power of these innovative treatments.

One impactful example involves a stroke survivor who had lost significant motor functions in her right arm. Through the dedicated use of constraint-induced movement therapy, a technique that involves restricting the use of her healthy arm to encourage the use of the affected one, she experienced remarkable progress. Over weeks, her brain adapted, developed new neural pathways, and restored a substantial degree of movement and functionality to her previously impaired limb.

Another case involved deep brain stimulation (DBS) for a patient suffering from severe Parkinson's disease. The patient struggled with tremors and bradykinesia that severely hindered daily activities. After undergoing DBS surgery where electrodes were implanted in specific brain areas, the patient saw a dramatic reduction in symptoms. This allowed him not only to perform daily tasks with much greater ease but also improved his overall quality of life significantly.

Furthermore, we consider the use of transcranial magnetic stimulation (TMS) in treating major depressive disorder. A patient, unresponsive to traditional antidepressants, turned to TMS. After several sessions where magnetic pulses were directed to stimulate her brain's frontal lobe, she reported a substantial improvement in mood and cognitive function, illustrating how TMS can serve as a lifeline for those with treatment-resistant depression.

These cases underscore the transformative potential of neuroplasticity-based therapies. By harnessing the brain's ability to reorganize itself, medical professionals are able to tailor treatments that offer real, observable benefits, effectively changing lives by restoring functions that once seemed irretrievably lost. This makes the role of neuroplasticity in modern medicine not just fascinating but truly life-altering.

The integration of neurotechnology into therapies presents both exciting possibilities and significant ethical considerations that must be addressed to ensure these advancements benefit everyone equitably. Neurotechnology, such as deep brain stimulation (DBS) and transcranial magnetic stimulation (TMS), offers groundbreaking potential in treating a range of neurological conditions from Parkinson's disease to depression. However, the deployment of such technologies raises critical questions concerning privacy, consent, and the potential for misuse.

For instance, while DBS can profoundly improve the quality of life for individuals with severe Parkinson's disease by controlling tremors, it involves implanting electrodes in the brain, which leads to concerns about the security of the neurological data collected. There's a necessity to protect this sensitive information from potential breaches that could expose personal health data. Furthermore, the irreversible nature of certain neurotechnological interventions requires informed consent processes that comprehensively cover potential risks and benefits, ensuring patients or their caregivers are fully aware and capable of making educated decisions.

Moreover, neurotechnology opens up discussions about the enhancement versus therapy dichotomy. Tools designed for therapeutic purposes might also be used for enhancing cognitive or physical capabilities in healthy individuals. This prospect invites debates on fairness, equity, and the societal implications of such enhancements. Who gets access to these technologies? And could this create a greater divide in a society where only those who can afford these costly treatments benefit from them?

Addressing these challenges requires robust ethical guidelines and regulatory frameworks that keep pace with technological advancements. Legislations need to be thoughtfully crafted and rigorously enforced to safeguard individual rights while fostering innovation. Dialogues between technologists, ethicists, legislators, and the greater public will be crucial in steering the development of neurotechnological therapies towards the most ethical and beneficial outcomes for society.

As these discussions unfold, it becomes imperative to remain vigilant about the motivations driving neurotechnological research and the deployment of its applications, ensuring that these powerful tools do not only serve a privileged few but contribute positively to the broad spectrum of society. The future of neurotechnology in therapy, therefore, not only promises immense medical advancements but also demands a careful, principled approach to its integration into healthcare and society.

The technological and therapeutic breakthroughs we've discussed have the potential to profoundly transform how neurological disorders are treated and how cognitive functions are enhanced. By leveraging advanced neurotechnologies like deep brain stimulation (DBS) and transcranial magnetic stimulation (TMS), coupled with innovative therapeutic strategies that harness the principles of neuroplasticity, medical professionals can offer more targeted, effective interventions.

These innovations enable a shift from traditional, often less specific treatment methods to personalized approaches that address the unique neural patterns of each patient. For instance, DBS provides targeted electrical stimulation to specific brain areas affected by disorders such as Parkinson's disease, significantly reducing symptoms and improving quality of life. Similarly, TMS has shown promising results in treating major depressive disorder by non-invasively modulating neural activity in specific cortical areas.

Moreover, the integration of artificial intelligence into these technologies enhances their effectiveness further. AI can analyze vast amounts of patient data to optimize treatment parameters in real-time, ensuring that each patient receives the most appropriate intervention. This adaptability not only improves immediate treatment outcomes but also contributes to long-term recovery and functionality.

In conclusion, these cutting-edge technologies and therapies not only pave the way for more effective treatment of neurological disorders but also push the boundaries of what is achievable in enhancing cognitive functions. As we continue to explore and refine these approaches, we open the door to a future where the treatment of neurological conditions is more precise, personalized, and impactful, ultimately leading to better patient outcomes and broader accessibility to high-quality care.

FUTURE DIRECTIONS IN NEUROPLASTICITY RESEARCH

The realm of neuroplasticity, the brain's remarkable ability to reorganize itself by forming new neural connections, stands on the brink of groundbreaking advancements. As researchers dive deeper into understanding this extraordinary feature of the human brain, they unveil potential that could revolutionize the treatment of neurological disorders and enhance cognitive functions dramatically. This burgeoning field of study not only promises significant therapeutic gains for ailments ranging from stroke recovery to mental health disorders but also offers insights into the everyday enhancements of brain function.

In this exploration of future directions in neuroplasticity research, we will uncover how the latest trends and emerging technologies are shaping our approach to brain health and recovery. Through precise methodology and clear elucidations, this chapter aims to illuminate the path forward in neuroscientific research, inviting you to understand and engage with the potentials that modern science is on the cusp of realizing. By providing a lucid breakdown of complex concepts and spotlighting their relevance in current and future applications, this introduction serves as your gateway into the dynamic and developing world of neuroplasticity. Whether you are a student, a healthcare professional, or simply a curious mind, the insights offered here are poised to enhance your comprehension of how flexible our brains truly are and the vast implications this holds for medical science and beyond.

The realm of neuroplasticity research continues to advance at an exhilarating pace, propelled by the advent of sophisticated technologies and methodologies. Among the prominent trends in this field, advanced neuroimaging techniques stand out for their ability to offer unprecedented views into the living brain. Techniques such as functional magnetic resonance imaging (fMRI) and positron emission tomography (PET) now allow researchers to observe neural activity in real-time, shedding light on how neuronal connections form and alter in response to various stimuli.

Parallel to imaging advancements, genetic research is unravelling how individual differences in genes affect the brain's potential to adapt. Pioneering studies are identifying specific genetic markers that influence neuroplasticity, providing insights that could lead to personalized therapy plans based on a person's genetic profile. This genetic mapping promises a future where treatments and cognitive therapies are finely tuned to one's genetic predispositions, optimizing the effectiveness of interventions aimed at harnessing neuroplasticity.

In the technological arena, enhancements in cognitive therapies are increasingly supported by tools such as virtual reality (VR) and augmented reality (AR). These technologies create immersive rehabilitation environments that can be precisely controlled and manipulated to stimulate brain activity in targeted ways. For example, a person recovering from a stroke might use a VR system programmed to provide activities that promote the rewiring of brain areas responsible for motor control and coordination.

Each of these trends contributes significantly to our expanding understanding of the brain's adaptability. By integrating findings from neuroimaging, genetic research, and technology-driven therapies, scientists are piecing together a more comprehensive picture of neuroplasticity. This intricate mosaic not only enriches our theoretical knowledge but also paves the way for practical applications that could transform how neurological disorders are treated, enhancing the lives of millions around the globe. This marriage of theory and application encapsulates the profound impact of current research trends on the field of neuroplasticity, promising a future where the brain's ability to adapt is harnessed to its fullest potential.

Let's take a deeper look at how advanced neuroimaging techniques like fMRI and PET contribute to our understanding of neuroplasticity, highlighting their specific roles, analysis, and contributions to the field.

Specific Capabilities:
Functional Magnetic Resonance Imaging (fMRI) and Positron Emission Tomography (PET) offer distinct insights into the brain's activity and plasticity. fMRI measures brain activity by detecting changes associated with blood flow, allowing researchers to see which areas of the brain are involved in specific mental processes. This is particularly useful in neuroplasticity studies for mapping how brain functions shift from one area to another after an injury. PET scans, on the other hand, use radioactive tracers

to visualize how specific substances, such as glucose, are metabolized in the brain. This can help in identifying how neural pathways are altered in response to changes in the brain's environment or condition.

Data Interpretation:
The data obtained from fMRI and PET scans are analyzed through various computational models that detect patterns of change over time. For fMRI, data analysis involves techniques such as voxel-based morphometry and functional connectivity analysis, which help elucidate the relationships between different brain regions and their co-activation patterns. PET data analysis often focuses on metabolic rates to infer neural activity levels, providing insight into the biochemical changes that underpin plasticity.

Direct Contributions to Neuroplasticity Research:
These imaging techniques have been pivotal in numerous studies. For example, fMRI has been extensively used to observe how the motor cortex reorganizes itself in stroke survivors undergoing rehabilitation. Similarly, PET scans have been instrumental in studying changes in brain metabolism in patients with Alzheimer's disease, offering clues about how synaptic connections deteriorate and potentially how they can be restored.

Comparative Analysis:
While both fMRI and PET provide valuable insights, they do so in different ways. fMRI offers greater spatial resolution, making it more effective for detailed anatomical mapping and understanding precise areas of activation. PET,

while generally lower in spatial resolution compared to fMRI, can provide unique insights into the chemical changes occurring in the brain, making it invaluable for studying neurotransmitter systems. These complementary strengths make fMRI and PET powerful tools for studying different aspects of neuroplasticity.

Interaction with Other Research Areas:
Findings from fMRI and PET are often integrated with genetic and cognitive therapy research to enhance our holistic understanding of neuroplasticity. Genetic research can elucidate why certain pathways are more susceptible to change, helping interpret imaging results within a broader genetic context. Conversely, insights from neuroimaging guide the development of targeted cognitive therapies by identifying specific brain areas that might benefit from intervention.

By dissecting how fMRI and PET contribute to neuroplasticity research, we can appreciate their invaluable role in advancing our understanding and treatment of brain disorders. This clarity deepens our appreciation of the complexities of brain function and the innovative tools we deploy to explore them, highlighting their relevance and impact on shaping future neurological healthcare.

Anticipated breakthroughs in neuroplastic therapies are poised to markedly improve treatments for neurological damage, cognitive impairments, and psychiatric disorders. These advancements harness the brain's intrinsic ability to reform and adapt, opening up new possibilities for recovery and enhancement that were once considered beyond reach.

One promising area involves the refinement of transcranial magnetic stimulation (TMS). Techniques are evolving to target specific brain regions more accurately, allowing for precise modulation of neural circuits involved in conditions like depression and schizophrenia. This precision could enhance the efficacy of TMS, reducing symptoms more effectively and rapidly than current treatments allow.

Similarly, developments in neurorehabilitation are leveraging augmented reality (AR) and virtual reality (VR) technology to create immersive therapy environments. For a patient recovering from a stroke, for instance, VR can simulate real-life tasks such as cooking or driving, providing a safe, controlled setting in which to regain motor skills and cognitive functions through repetitive practice. These activities are designed to stimulate specific neural pathways, encouraging the brain to rewire itself and regain lost capabilities.

In the realm of cognitive impairments, advances in our understanding of neuroplasticity are leading to targeted cognitive training approaches. For individuals with Alzheimer's disease, new therapies are under development that aim to slow the progression of symptoms by reinforcing neural connectivity and function in affected regions of the brain. These therapies often employ computer-based exercises that adapt to the user's performance, maintaining an optimal level of challenge and engagement to foster brain adaptability.

Mapping the impact of these neuroplastic therapies offers an intricate view of how targeted interventions can coax the brain into making functional adjustments. These therapies not only hold potential for greater recovery rates but also promise a future where psychiatric and neurological care is vastly more personalized and effective.

As we dive deeper into the nuances of these therapies, it becomes evident that the road ahead is filled with innovative approaches that could redefine our expectations for treating brain-related disorders. These advancements underline the importance of continued research and funding in neuroplasticity, ensuring these emerging therapies reach their full potential and become accessible to those in need.

Step 1: Overview of Neuroplasticity

Neuroplasticity refers to the brain's capacity to reorganize itself by forming new neural connections throughout life. This ability is crucial because it underpins the brain's adaptation to learning, experiences, and even recovery from injuries. Understanding neuroplasticity forms the foundation for developing innovative treatments that leverage the brain's inherent adaptability, offering new ways to mitigate and rehabilitate neurological and psychiatric conditions.

Step 2: Mechanisms of TMS

Transcranial Magnetic Stimulation (TMS) is a non-invasive method used to modulate neuronal activity. It involves placing a magnetic coil near the skull, where it generates focused magnetic pulses. These pulses induce electric fields that stimulate specific areas of the brain. The key to TMS is the precise targeting of these regions, often identified through neuroimaging techniques that map the brain's functional areas related to specific disorders, such as depression or motor rehabilitation after a stroke.

Step 3: Application of VR in Rehabilitation

Virtual Reality (VR) is employed in rehabilitation to create controlled, immersive environments tailored to individual therapeutic needs. These VR settings simulate real-life challenges that patients need to master again, like walking, driving, or even complex hand movements. The design of these tasks is based on a patient's specific deficits and the neuroplastic goals of therapy, such as enhancing motor control or improving spatial awareness, thereby stimulating the reorganization of relevant neural pathways in the brain.

Step 4: Cognitive Training for Cognitive Impairments

Cognitive training utilizes computer-based exercises designed to improve cognitive functions by strengthening neural connectivity. These programs are adaptive; they scale in difficulty in response to user performance, ensuring the brain is sufficiently challenged. For instance, tasks may be designed to enhance memory, speed of processing, or problem-solving skills in individuals with cognitive impairments like Alzheimer's disease. The tailoring of tasks to specific neural deficits is central to the success of these interventions.

Step 5: Integration and Personalization

In practice, data from TMS, VR rehabilitation, and

cognitive training sessions are continuously gathered and analyzed. This analysis helps in fine-tuning the interventions to better suit individual patient needs and progress. Machine learning algorithms can be used to predict which types of adjustments in therapeutic regimes might yield better outcomes based on ongoing data, leading to increasingly personalized treatment plans.

Step 6: The Future of Neuroplastic Therapies

Looking forward, the field of neuroplastic therapies is likely to see significant advancements that further customize and enhance treatment efficacy. Continued research might bring about more sophisticated neuromodulation techniques, deeper integration with real-time neuroimaging, and smarter AI-driven therapy systems that can predict and adapt to a patient's unique brain activity patterns even more effectively. The ongoing commitment to research and innovation is essential for realizing these potentials, ensuring that future treatments can be even more targeted and effective.

This step-by-step guide outlines how cutting-edge developments in neuroplastic therapies are being practically applied to revolutionize the treatment landscape for patients with neurological and psychiatric issues, heralding a future where such conditions are managed more effectively than ever before.

Advancing neuroplasticity research brings forth a myriad of complexities and ethical dilemmas that need careful consideration, particularly in areas like patient consent, artificial intelligence integration, and brain-computer interfacing. Let's dissect these complex elements to better understand the challenges and responsibilities involved.

Starting with patient consent, it's crucial in neuroplasticity research where experimental treatments or technologies might be employed. Gaining informed consent involves more than just a signature; it necessitates that patients are thoroughly informed about the potential risks, benefits, and unknowns of participating in studies that manipulate brain activity. Researchers must ensure that information is communicated in a manner that is understandable to patients without minimizing the risks or exaggerating the potential benefits.

Turning to the use of artificial intelligence (AI), this technology plays a significant role in analyzing vast amounts of data from neuroplasticity experiments and in predicting outcomes of neural interventions. However, the incorporation of AI also introduces concerns about data privacy and algorithmic bias. The sensitive nature of neurodata makes it imperative that stringent measures are put in place to protect patient information from misuse or breaches. Additionally, biases in AI algorithms can lead to skewed research outcomes or discriminatory therapeutic practices, highlighting the need for ongoing scrutiny and calibration of AI systems used in research.

Brain-computer interfacing (BCI) represents another area padded with ethical questions. BCIs literally connect human thoughts with external devices, offering revolutionary possibilities for individuals with severe disabilities by enabling control over prosthetics or computers through neural activity alone. Nevertheless, this groundbreaking technology stirs debates about identity, autonomy, and consent, especially concerning individuals whose cognitive impairments might limit their understanding or ability to give informed consent. Furthermore, long-term impacts on individuals' neurological health and psychological well-being remain largely uncharted, requiring a cautious and reflective approach to development and implementation.

Each of these elements underscores the need to balance innovation with ethical responsibility. As researchers push the boundaries of what's possible in neuroplasticity, it's vital to maintain rigorous ethical standards to ensure that the pursuits do not inadvertently harm those they aim to help. This deep dive into the complexities and ethical dilemmas encourages a dialogue that is as much about scientific exploration as it is about maintaining humanity's moral compass in uncharted territories.

Here is the detailed breakdown of the ethical concerns and mitigation strategies related to the use of artificial intelligence in neuroplasticity research:

- **Data Privacy**:
  - **Risk Assessment**:
    - **Types of Data Collected**: Typically includes personal health information, brain imaging data, and possibly genetic data which are highly sensitive.
    - **Potential Vulnerabilities**: Risks may include unauthorized access, data breaches, and unintended data sharing.

- **Risks to Patient Privacy**: Breaches could lead to privacy violations and damage to patient trust and confidence in the medical system.
  - **Protection Measures**:
    - **Encryption**: Employing strong encryption methods while storing and transmitting data to prevent unauthorized access.
    - **Access Control**: Implementing strict access controls and authentication measures to ensure only authorized personnel can access sensitive data.
    - **Cybersecurity Measures**: Regular audits, updating security protocols, and training staff in cybersecurity best practices to safeguard data.

- **Algorithmic Bias**:
  - **Source of Bias**:
    - **Training Data Selection**: If the data used to train AI algorithms are not diverse, they may not perform well across different populations.
    - **Algorithm Design**: Flaws in algorithm design could inadvertently introduce bias.
  - **Impact on Research and Therapy**:
    - **Research Outcomes**: Bias can lead to inaccurate conclusions about neuroplasticity, potentially affecting the validity of the research.
    - **Therapeutic Applications**: Biased algorithms may lead to unequal treatment effectiveness, affecting certain groups disproportionately.
  - **Preventive Actions**:
    - **Algorithm Auditing**: Regular reviews and audits of algorithms to identify and correct bias.
    - **Diversified Data Training Sets**: Using diverse data sets that represent different populations to train algorithms,

ensuring they are effective across diverse groups.

- **Regulatory Compliance and Oversight**:
  - **Existing Regulations**:
    - **General Data Protection Regulation (GDPR)**: European regulation that provides guidelines for the collection and processing of personal information.
    - **Health Insurance Portability and Accountability Act (HIPAA)**: US legislation that provides data privacy and security provisions for safeguarding medical information.
  - **Compliance Strategies**:
    - **Monitoring and Reporting**: Establishing systems for continuous monitoring of compliance and mechanisms for reporting violations promptly.
    - **Adhering to Ethical Standards**: Ensuring that all AI applications in research adhere to established ethical standards and guidelines.

- **Ethic Committees and Reviews**:
  - **Role of Institutional Review Boards (IRBs)**: IRBs review research proposals to ensure that they are ethically sound and that participants are not subjected to unnecessary risk.
  - **Ethics Committees**:
    - **Oversight**: Monitoring ongoing projects to ensure they comply with ethical standards throughout the research cycle.

This comprehensive outline sheds light on the key ethical considerations and strategies for mitigating risks associated with AI in neuroplasticity research. By addressing these issues proactively, researchers can ensure that their work not only advances scientific knowledge but also upholds the highest ethical standards, reinforcing the integrity of neuroscientific advancements.

Imagine you're upgrading the operating system on your smartphone. This upgrade improves the phone's performance and even allows it to learn from your usage patterns to enhance battery efficiency or application responses. This closely mirrors the principles behind neuroplasticity research, where scientists develop therapies that essentially upgrade the brain's 'operating system' to enhance its functions and enable recovery from injuries.

For instance, just as a smartphone learns to open your most used apps quicker, neuroplastic therapy can train the brain to reroute functions taken over by damaged areas to healthy regions, improving recovery in stroke survivors. Think of it as your phone reassigning its resources to maintain functionality when one part stops working, like using a cloud service when the internal memory fails.

In practical terms, this research translates into real-world treatments like physical therapy aided by virtual reality. Just as pilots simulate flights in their training, stroke survivors can use VR platforms to practice and regain everyday skills in a controlled environment, continually improving through repetition—much like playing a video game where you advance with each level conquered.

Furthermore, cognitive training apps, inspired by puzzle-solving games, leverage neuroplasticity to slow cognitive decline in aging populations or in conditions like Alzheimer's. Each puzzle solved or level passed is similar to strengthening a neural pathway, helping the brain stay 'in shape' much like a daily crossword keeps one's vocabulary sharp.

Understanding neuroplasticity through these everyday analogies not only highlights how deeply interwoven it is with familiar experiences but also underscores its importance in advancing medical science and enhancing lives. This field's ongoing research is not merely academic—it's a promising frontier with tangible benefits, potentially as impactful as the smartphone revolution, bringing theoretical insights into concrete, personal gains.

To deepen understanding and spark curiosity about neuroplasticity, consider engaging with the following ChatGPT prompts within ChatGPT. This will help your understand as each prompt is designed to explore different facets of neuroplasticity, encouraging a conversational approach that makes complex scientific concepts more digestible and engaging:

1. **"Explain neuroplasticity in simple terms."**
Use this prompt to have ChatGPT break down the concept of neuroplasticity into basic, easily understandable language. It's a great starting point for those new to the topic.

2. **"How does neuroplasticity change as we age?"**

This prompt encourages ChatGPT to discuss the effects of aging on the brain's ability to rewire itself. It will explore changes from childhood through to old age, providing insights into why certain periods are critical for cognitive development.

3. "Give examples of how neuroplasticity is involved in recovery from brain injuries."

Here, ChatGPT can explain how neuroplasticity is leveraged in therapeutic settings, particularly in the rehabilitation of patients with brain injuries like strokes or traumatic brain injuries.

4. "Describe a day in the life of someone undergoing neuroplastic therapy."

This creative prompt helps users visualize the practical application of neuroplastic therapies by narrating a patient's daily routine, thereby connecting high-level concepts with personal human experiences.

5. "What role does technology play in advancing our understanding of neuroplasticity?"

Ask ChatGPT to outline current technological tools like fMRI or TMS and discuss how these are used in neuroplastic research and therapies, highlighting the bridge between technology and neuroscience.

6. "Can lifestyle changes influence neuroplasticity? Provide practical tips."

This prompt dives into how everyday activities and choices can affect the brain's plasticity. ChatGPT can offer advice on habits that promote brain health, such as diet, exercise, and mental challenges.

7. "Discuss the ethical considerations in neuroplasticity research."

Engage ChatGPT in a deeper conversation about the ethical dilemmas faced by researchers working with brain intervention technologies, focusing on issues such as consent and the potential long-term effects of brain manipulation.

8. "Predict future trends in neuroplastic research and their potential impact on society."

This forward-looking prompt invites ChatGPT to speculate on future developments in neuroplasticity, such as personalized brain enhancement, and discuss their implications for education, healthcare, and daily life.

These prompts are structured to facilitate a deeper understanding and appreciation of neuroplasticity. They aim to illuminate not just the scientific basis but also the broader implications and applications of this dynamic field, enhancing engagement in a way that resonates with personal experiences and current societal contexts.

Here are some ChatGPT Prompts that revolve around exploring and understanding neuroplasticity:

[**Understanding Neuroplasticity Through Everyday Activities**] - **Objective**: This prompt is designed to help users relate the concept of neuroplasticity to everyday activities to understand its impact on daily life.

- **Prompt**: "Explain how daily activities like learning a new language or playing a musical instrument can enhance neuroplasticity."

- **Sample Output**: "Engaging in activities that challenge your brain, like learning a new language or playing an instrument, helps to form new neural connections. This process, known as neuroplasticity, improves various cognitive functions such as memory, attention, and problem-solving skills."

- **Follow Up**: Reflect on the explanation and think of personal experiences where you might have witnessed neuroplasticity without realizing it.

[Debating Ethical Concerns in Neuroplasticity Enhancements] - **Objective**: To draw attention to and foster discussion on the ethical decisions involved in applying neuroplasticity research, especially concerning cognitive enhancements.

- **Prompt**: "Discuss the ethical implications of using neuroplasticity-enhancing technologies for non-medical purposes, such as improving cognitive abilities in healthy individuals."

- **Sample Output**: "The use of neuroplasticity-enhancing technologies raises significant ethical questions. One concern is equity—whether these technologies would only be available to those who can afford them, potentially widening social inequalities. Another issue is long-term safety, which remains largely unknown."

- **Follow Up**: Consider the ethical implications discussed and formulate your stance on this issue. Engage in a debate or discussion forum to explore diverse perspectives.

[**Predicting the Future of Neuroplasticity Research**] - **Objective**: Encourage users to think critically about how the future of neuroplasticity research could look and its potential societal impacts.

- **Prompt**: "Predict how neuroplasticity research might evolve over the next two decades and discuss its potential impacts on how we treat neurological disorders."

- **Sample Output**: "In the next twenty years, neuroplasticity research could lead to highly personalized brain rehabilitation techniques that cater to the specific neural wiring of each patient, significantly improving recovery rates from brain injuries. Additionally, advancements in this field might help prevent or delay the onset of neurodegenerative diseases."

- **Follow Up**: Use this prediction to research current trends in neuroplasticity and view how they might evolve. Consider writing an article or blog post on your thoughts and findings.

[**Exploring Neuroplasticity in Learning and Memory**] - **Objective**: To understand the role of neuroplasticity in learning new skills and forming memories.

- **Prompt**: "Describe how neuroplasticity is involved in the process of learning a new skill and forming memories."

- **Sample Output**: "Neuroplasticity plays a crucial role in learning and memory. When you learn a new skill, your brain changes structurally and functionally; neurons form new connections, strengthening pathways that are frequently used, which helps in forming and retaining new memories related to the skill."

- **Follow Up**: Apply this knowledge to a new skill you are learning, and observe how consistent practice and exposure enhance your proficiency over time.

[Neuroplasticity and Recovery from Trauma]
- **Objective**: Investigate how mechanisms of neuroplasticity contribute to recovery from traumatic brain injuries or psychological trauma.
- **Prompt**: "Explain how neuroplasticity assists in the recovery process from traumatic brain injuries and psychological trauma."
- **Sample Output**: "Neuroplasticity facilitates recovery by allowing the brain to rewire itself and compensate for injured areas. This is achieved through various rehabilitation exercises that encourage the formation of new neural pathways, gradually restoring lost functions and helping individuals recover from trauma."
- **Follow Up**: If applicable, explore case studies or research papers that illustrate real-life recovery stories enabled by neuroplasticity, underlining the practical benefits of this incredible brain capability.

[Harnessing Neuroplasticity for Stress Management]
- **Objective**: To explore how neuroplasticity can be utilized in everyday stress management strategies.
- **Prompt**: "Discuss how regular meditation or mindfulness practices can leverage neuroplasticity for better stress management."
- **Sample Output**: "Regular engagement in meditation or mindfulness practices can enhance neuroplasticity by strengthening neural pathways associated with self-regulation and calmness. Over time, these practices help the brain to become more efficient at managing stress, reducing the overall psychological and physical impact of stressors."
- **Follow Up**: Implement a regular meditation or mindfulness routine and note any changes in your stress

levels and general well-being over a period of time.

[Neuroplasticity in Child Development and Learning] - **Objective**: To understand the role of neuroplasticity in child development and learning processes.
   - **Prompt**: "Explain how neuroplasticity influences child development, particularly in the context of learning new cognitive and motor skills."
   - **Sample Output**: "During childhood, the brain's neuroplasticity is at its peak, which facilitates rapid learning and development. This plastic nature allows young brains to easily form new connections, which is crucial for acquiring language skills, solving problems, and developing fine motor skills necessary for writing and drawing."
   - **Follow Up**: Observe and document learning behaviors in children, such as how quickly they pick up new languages or adapt to new physical activities, to see neuroplasticity in action.

[Impact of Nutrition on Neuroplasticity] - **Objective**: To analyze how nutrition affects the brain's plasticity and overall cognitive health.
   - **Prompt**: "Discuss the impact of essential nutrients like Omega-3 fatty acids on brain plasticity and cognitive functions."
   - **Sample Output**: "Omega-3 fatty acids, found in foods like fish, flaxseeds, and walnuts, play a crucial role in maintaining and enhancing neuroplasticity. They are vital components of neuronal membranes and help in the formation of new neural connections, significantly impacting learning, memory, and cognitive speed."
   - **Follow Up**: Adjust your diet to include a higher intake

of Omega-3-rich foods and monitor any noticeable changes in your cognitive abilities.

[Neuroplasticity and Aging: Strategies to Maintain Cognitive Health] - **Objective**: To identify practices that older adults can adopt to promote neuroplasticity as they age.
  - **Prompt**: "Provide strategies that can help maintain or even improve neuroplasticity in the aging population."
  - **Sample Output**: "Engaging in regular physical exercise, continuous learning activities, and social interactions are effective strategies for older adults to promote brain plasticity. Such activities help maintain cognitive functions and may delay the onset of age-related cognitive decline."
  - **Follow Up**: If applicable, involve an older adult in these activities, track their progress over time, and note any improvements in cognitive functions or overall mental health.

[The Interplay Between Neuroplasticity and Sleep] - **Objective**: To dive into how sleep influences neuroplasticity and the consolidation of new memories.
  - **Prompt**: "Explain the relationship between sleep and neuroplasticity, particularly focusing on memory consolidation."
  - **Sample Output**: "Sleep plays a critical role in neuroplasticity, particularly in the consolidation of memories. During sleep, especially during deep REM phases, the brain processes and integrates new knowledge and experiences into long-term memory, thereby strengthening new neural connections."
  - **Follow Up**: Analyze your own sleep patterns and their

correlation with learning or memory retention. Try adjusting sleep habits to optimize memory consolidation and observe the outcomes.

By engaging with the range of ChatGPT prompts provided, you will gain a comprehensive understanding of neuroplasticity's profound influence across various dimensions of human life. These prompts are crafted to explore neuroplasticity's fundamental principles and its practical applications in fields such as therapeutic interventions, cognitive well-being, child development, aging, and overall lifestyle impacts. Utilizing these prompts enables you to grasp how neuroplastic mechanisms are pivotal in recovery from neurological damage, how they evolve with aging, and how everyday activities can enhance cognitive flexibility. This detailed journey through different scenarios and explanations will not only broaden your comprehension but also equip you with actionable knowledge that can be applied in personal health strategies or in supporting others in your community. Through a simplified yet thorough exploratory process, you'll witness the possibilities of enhancing brain function and maintaining cognitive health via lifestyle choices, innovative therapies, and more.

In executing all these prompts, you will achieve:

- **Enhanced Knowledge**: Deepen your understanding of how neuroplasticity functions and affects various life stages and conditions.

- **Practical Insights**: Gain actionable insights into how lifestyle choices, therapeutic practices, and educational strategies can influence neuroplasticity.

- **Ethical Awareness**: Develop a nuanced perspective of the ethical considerations in neuroplastic technologies and therapies.
- **Future Foresight**: Explore potential future developments in neuroplasticity research and their implications for society and individual well-being.
- **Personal Connection**: Link the concepts of neuroplasticity to personal or observed experiences, making the knowledge more tangible and applicable.
- **Community Benefit**: Equip yourself with information and strategies that can benefit not just personal health but also contribute to community awareness and wellness initiatives.

This chapter has intricately laid out the pivotal role of neuroplasticity research in transforming our approach to neurological health, illustrating both the immediate benefits and the far-reaching potential it holds for future medical treatments. Neuroplasticity, the brain's ability to rewire and adapt, stands at the forefront of revolutionary treatment strategies for an array of neurological and psychiatric conditions. Innovations such as neurorehabilitative therapies using virtual reality, enhanced cognitive training methods, and advanced neuroimaging techniques have all been shown to significantly improve outcomes for patients with conditions ranging from traumatic brain injuries to Alzheimer's disease.

Each facet of the discussed neuroplasticity advancements contributes to a broader understanding and more effective application of therapeutic practices, emphasizing the adaptability and resilience of the human brain. The integration of artificial intelligence and machine learning further magnifies the scope and precision of neuroplastic treatments, offering customized therapeutic approaches tailored to individual neural patterns of patients.

Crucially, the ethical dimensions surrounding the use of emerging neuroplastic technologies have been acknowledged and addressed, ensuring that the march towards innovation does not outpace the consideration of moral implications. As this research progresses, it not only promises to refine our current treatment paradigms but also paves the way for preventative strategies that could mitigate the onset of neurological deterioration.

By continuing to support and expand neuroplasticity research, the potential to enhance life quality for millions around the globe is immense. This is not merely theoretical; it's a tangible path forward in medicine that beckons with prospects of recovery and rejuvenation of neural functions, fundamentally altering the landscape of neurological healthcare.

CONCLUSION

As we conclude our exploration in "Neuroplasticity Explained," it's evident that the brain's ability to adapt and reshape itself is one of the most extraordinary aspects of human biology. Through the pages of this book, we've journeyed from the fundamental principles of neuroplasticity to the cutting-edge research that continues to push the boundaries of what we understand about the brain's capacity for change.

We have learned that neuroplasticity is not just a response to injury but a constant feature of a healthy brain, engaging in the background of everyday activities such as learning new skills, forming memories, or even navigating complex social interactions. The lessons on how lifestyle choices like exercise, diet, and continuous learning impact our brain plasticity are both empowering and a call to action. These insights underscore the proactive role we can all play in enhancing our cognitive health and overall well-being.

Reflecting on the broader implications, this book highlights neuroplasticity's significant role in clinical settings, particularly in rehabilitation from brain injuries and in the treatment of neurological disorders. The potential for future therapies that harness this inherent adaptability of the brain opens up hopeful prospects for millions of individuals affected by such conditions.

"Neuroplasticity Explained" has also introduced complex theories and current debates within the scientific community, challenging us to think critically about the ethical dimensions of neuroplastic research and its applications. As we stand on the cusp of technological advancements that could redefine human potential, these discussions are more relevant than ever.

Leaving you with final thoughts to ponder, I encourage you to consider how the plastic nature of the brain not only embodies our capacity for resilience and recovery but also reflects our profound interconnectedness with our environments and each other. The science of neuroplasticity, much like the brain itself, is not just about individual neurons or specific techniques; it's about the broader networks and the dynamic interactions that shape our experiences and our selves.

As you turn the last page of this book, may your understanding of neuroplasticity not only enrich your appreciation of human biology but also inspire a lifelong curiosity about the untapped potentials that reside within your own neural pathways.

ABOUT THE AUTHOR

Alex Rossi brings a wealth of experience from over twenty years in the information technology industry, having worked with some of the world's leading tech giants.

With a deep-seated passion for science, technology, and languages, Alex excels at demystifying complex subjects, making them accessible and engaging to a broad audience. His writings focus on breaking down intricate topics into everyday terms, helping readers not just learn but also apply this knowledge in their daily lives.

Currently, Alex is a proud member of Green Mountain Publishing, which publishes his insightful books. Through his work, he aims to foster a deeper understanding and appreciation of technology and science, enriching readers' lives.

Printed in Great Britain
by Amazon